Playing the Game

A Step-by-Step Approach to Accepting Insurance as an Acupuncturist

by Dr. Greg Sperber
& Tiffany Andersen-Hefner

Published by:
BLUE POPPY PRESS
A Division of Blue Poppy Enterprises, Inc.
1990 N 57th Court, Unit A
BOULDER, CO 80301
www.bluepoppy.com

First Printing, September, 2011
Second Printing, March, 2014
Third Printing, February, 2015

ISBN 1-891845-59-4
ISBN 978-1-891845-59-8
LCCN #2011910171

COPYRIGHT © BLUE POPPY PRESS, 2011. All Rights Reserved.

All rights reserved. No part of this book may be reproduced, stored in a retrieval system, transcribed in any form or by any means, electronic, mechanical, photocopy, recording, or any other means, or translated into any language without the prior written permission of the publisher.

DISCLAIMER: The information in this book is given in good faith. However, the author and the publishers cannot be held responsible for any error or omission. The publishers will not accept liabilities for any injuries or damages caused to the reader that may result from the reader's acting upon or using the content contained in this book. The publishers make this information available to English language readers for research and scholarly purposes only.

The publishers do not advocate nor endorse self-medication by laypersons. Chinese medicine is a professional medicine. Laypersons interested in availing themselves of the treatments described in this book should seek out a qualified professional practitioner of Chinese medicine.

COMP Designation: Compilation of functional translations using a standard translational terminology plus an original work.

Page layout design by Deborah Topping, Honora Lee Wolfe; and composed by Eric J. Brearton
Cover design by Eric J. Brearton, cover illustration by Tom Johnson

10 9 8 7 6 5 4 3

Printed at Edwards Brothers Malloy, Ann Arbor, MI, on recycled paper and soy inks.

Insurance is a game.
Insurance has rules.
You have to play by their rules.

Insurance companies want to pay,
As long as you play by the rules.

Marilyn Allen

Table of Contents

6. After the Patient Leaves 109

7. Daily, Weekly, Monthly, and Yearly Annual Insurance Procedures 125

Acknowledgments

Putting together a book is never just the hard work of the authors. Many people, knowingly or otherwise, participate in the endeavor.

We would like to thank our families for allowing us the space, freedom, support, and, most importantly, the time to pursue this little work. To this end, thank you Leo Hefner, Maile Hefner, Bianca Baribeau, Diane Sperber, Marv Mittleman, Katie Sperber-Olguin, and Estelle Rosten. Mrs. Andersen-Hefner would especially like to thank Dr. Allyn Cano-Alwa for being an inspiration and setting her path to the acupuncture profession.

Thank you to those who helped us gather the technical knowledge to make this possible including Marilyn Allen, Sam Collins, and Shawn Steele. And to Starbucks who gave us the space and fuel to write.

And finally, thank you to the staff at Blue Poppy, especially Honora Lee Wolfe, who patiently awaited our manuscript, guided it through the arduous editing process, and printed the wonderful book the reader holds in their hand(s).

Warning

Things change rapidly in insurance. And they change slowly in publishing. Especially given the recent passage of healthcare reform, there may be rapid and dramatic changes to how healthcare is paid for in this country and what role acupuncture may play. Therefore, there may be many things in this book that change. As authors we promise do our best to include changes in book revisions, in addendums to the book, and especially on our website: **www.acu-insurance.com**, which you should check often. From the website, sign up for our email list, so you can be informed as rapidly as possible of any changes. Lastly, the authors and publisher have attempted to give the most up to date and comprehensive information available and are not responsible or liable for any damages resulting from the use of any information derived from this book. It is the reader's responsibility to verify the contents and remain current on any changes in the insurance system.

Introduction

This book started from several interesting happenings. When a new practice owner who needed to develop procedures for accepting insurance was introduced to an individual who had been an insurance biller for 12 years, this book was conceived. As we talked, there was a lot of agreement about what was missing from the literature in the Oriental medical field with regards to practice organization, administration and billing/collections procedures. And we both just really wanted to help acupuncturists be more successful.

As we wrote the book, we came across many standard difficulties including how to organize it, what should be included, and how to say what we wanted in a way that was easy to understand and implement. One of the important things we thought about was how to portray insurance. As we talked about it, we realized that insurance is something of a game. Sometimes you lose, but most of the time you win, maybe not as much as hoped, but still a win. If acupuncturists took this approach, maybe the whole insurance thing would be less daunting and more approachable. So we decided to call it The Game.

As in any game you need a playing field, rules, and the right equipment. We will explore all three of these throughout the book. We define the rules as not only how to get paid, but how to maximize your payments. The playing field is the regulatory and legal landscape as well as the arbitrary restrictions of the insurance companies. And the equipment is exactly that: what you need in order to be as efficient as possible as well as what may be required in the near future.

In this introduction, we will start to define the playing field by looking at what insurance is and the different types of insurance.

What is insurance?

Before delving into the different types of insurance, the actual role of insurance should be discussed. At its heart, insurance of all stripes is a risk management tool. It is designed to minimize the risk of having a catastrophe wipe out a family's or business' financial wherewithal. Hence we have fire insurance to protect a home or business from a random catastrophe from which it would be financially very hard to recover. So thousands or millions of people pay into a central pool of money and for the few that do have a disaster occur, they can recover and move on. In essence, it is a numbers game. A large number of people pay a small amount so that a few can receive a large amount and recover. It is a win-win-win situation. An individual pays a small amount of money to protect against a disaster, someone or some entity that does have a disaster befall them can continue to survive and prosper, and a company brokering all this can make some money, in an ideal world.

In reality, you have companies that want to make ever larger profits, catastrophes that do not follow set patterns (how dare they), and onerous rules about distribution. However, it would be very hard for anyone living in the United States or other first-world nations to avoid having any insurance. In most states, acupuncturists are required to have malpractice insurance. Drivers are mandated to have car insurance. And of course, there is health insurance. In most first-world nations, health insurance is administered and controlled by the government. In the United States, it is run by companies, both those that offer select options to their employees and other companies that administer it.

Health insurance is said to have begun with the Massachusetts Health Insurance of Boston in 1847, but was rudimentary when compared with health insurance today. Most insurance policies of the 1800s only covered accidents during travel. The first modern insurance policy is considered to have occurred in 1929 when a group of Dallas teachers contracted with Baylor Hospital. This rapidly increased in the 1930s and 40s. Blue Cross and Blue Shield began to form in 1932. In conjunction with this is the rise of biomedicine. Until the mid 1800s, medicine was abysmal; you had a higher chance of dying if you entered the medical system than if you did not. As modern biomedicine became more established and sophisticated, its costs became more onerous. Unions looking to increase benefits for members and businesses trying to recruit candidates also sparked a dramatic increase in demand during the mid 1900s. In the 1980s and 90s, technology rapidly increased the costs of medicine and insurance companies tried to control these costs by introducing managed care plans.

Today, there are a wide variety of health insurance options in the United States. Clamoring for a national healthcare system is stronger than ever. The one thing that the history of health insurance tells the observer is that rapid change is a constant. Health insurance at its most basic is a very useful tool for preventing catastrophe to our bank accounts. Whether it actually helps our health is another discussion.

Types of insurance

There are many different types of insurance. Each type needs to be approached differently by acupuncturists and has pros and cons to dealing with them. In general, having a diverse practice shields a provider from the vicissitudes of the economy and regulatory changes.

Health Maintenance Organizations (HMOs)

A Health Maintenance Organization (HMO) is a managed care company that provides comprehensive medical services to an enrolled population usually paid by using capitation. Capitation means that enrolled individuals or their employers pay a Per Member Per Month rate (PMPM) or a monthly fee per person. This means the HMO assumes the risk of a population overutilizing services and costing more than what was paid to the company. Individuals usually pay a small copay for each medical service while the HMO pays the rest.

HMOs come in two types: staff model and the group practice model. Staff model HMOs are those where the HMO owns the hospitals and other facilities in their system and hires the medical providers as employees to provide care for the enrollees. The prime example of this in the United States is Kaiser Permanente.

The group practice model HMOs are where individual hospitals and other facilities and medical providers, either individually or in groups, contract with an insurance company to provide medical services to patients. The providers are not considered employees and are free to contract with whomever they wish.

In either type of HMO, it is almost impossible to be reimbursed for services if a provider is not directly or indirectly contracted with the HMO. Even then, most services, including acupuncture, must be preapproved by a primary care physician (PCP). The PCP is often called the "gatekeeper" in an HMO system and all medical complaints must first be discussed with him or her and then either treated by them or referred out for more appropriate treatment. The thought is that a PCP, acting as a gatekeeper, can reduce the costs involved with unnecessary referrals.

General Insurance or Fee-for-service (FFS)

Up until the 1980s–90s, insurance was fee-for-service (FFS). This system gives the patient much of the control over which medical provider they go to and why. They pay a small percent of the services while the insurance company pays the rest after a deductible is met. A deductible is a dollar amount where the patient pays 100% of covered services up to a certain amount before the insurance kicks in. While varying greatly over the years, today a deductible is usually between $250-1,000 or $1,500+ for a high deductible plan. In a typical FFS plan, the patient would pay 20% of the fee with the insurance company paying 80%.

In the past, these plans were very lucrative for medical providers because there was not a lot of review of their services and they could bill as often and as much as they wanted. Today, they are subject to usual, customary, and reasonable (UCR) restrictions to their charges and utilization review is more stringent. However, they do tend to be among the easiest forms of insurance to work with, even as an acupuncturist. They are also among the rarest of insurance plans today.

Preferred Provider Organizations (PPOs)

Preferred provider organizations (PPOs) are sort of a cross between HMO and FFS insurance plans. While they offer the freedom of going to any medical provider the patient prefers, the patient will pay considerably more by going to a provider that is not contracted with the insurance plan, whereas they can save more by going to a preferred provider. This allows the company to reduce their costs and apply some restrictions as an HMO would, but still provide some of the freedom of an FFS plan. Cost is also somewhere in between the two plans. Acupuncturists can usually do well within a PPO plan, but they need to look at differences between being contracted or out-of-network (see Chapter 1).

Health Savings Accounts (HSAs)

Health savings accounts (HSAs) are a different breed of insurance altogether. They allow an individual to put pretax dollars into a savings account to help pay for health care costs. They combine this with a high-deductible insurance plan to cover catastrophic medical needs. Over time, this account can become quite large. They can also be used for retirement. In addition, depending on the company, HSAs offer, by far, the most freedom in what the account can be used for. In fact, this is the only insurance product that *may* cover the cost of prescribed herbs. Currently these are gaining popularity and, since they do offer the most for Oriental medical practitioners, as a profession we should be promoting them.

Health Reimbursement Accounts (HRAs)

Health Reimbursement Accounts (HRAs) are similar to an HSA but it is the employer who conributes a predetermined amount to an individual's account annually. These funds can be used to pay for medical care. Covered expenses are paid from the HRA at 100% (or a percentage determined by the employer) until the HRA balance is exhausted.

Typically when billing insurance, after the charges are processed, any patient portions would automatically get paid by any available HRA monies. Usually, once this fund is exhausted, the member is responsible for any remaining deductible charges or co-pays. An explanation of benefits would normally say that, if there are any available funds in the patient's HRA, payment will be forthcoming. The existence of an HRA is typically stated during an insurance verification.

Self-funded Plans

Self-funded plans technically can be any of the above types of insurance. They are instituted by very large companies who want to save money by not paying for insurance by an outside company. They basically fund their own in house insurance company. However, since they are not insurance companies, they do hire insurance companies to administer their plans. Often, for example, a patient will have a Blue Cross card, but the plan itself is not Blue Cross' but their employer's. Whichever type of insurance the company chooses to offer dictates how they will pay for acupuncture. But there is one way where they differ dramatically from the other types of insurance discussed: parity laws.

Parity laws in some states, including California, that say if an insurance company pays for acupuncture if a medical doctor performs it, they must pay the same if an acupuncturist performs it. But since a self-funded company is not an insurance company and is created under federal law, they are almost always exempt from parity laws. In other words, they can pay an M.D. but not an acupuncturist for providing acupuncture. Another exception to a state's parity law is federal insurance plans. This is because a state cannot enact laws that can change federal laws or regulations. Only a handful of states currently have parity laws, but several states are trying to enact them. They are beneficial for our profession and every practitioner should join their state and national professional organizations so we can pursue these and other laws that protect and promote acupuncture.

Workers' Compensation (WC)

Workers' compensation (WC) plans are required by most states to cover accidents and injuries that occur in the workplace or due to performing one's duties as an employee. Generally they resemble fee-for-service plans though they usually have an onerous and strict utilization review process which can include preapproval, elaborate relationships both between the practitioners and the WC insurance carriers as well as between practitioners. In California and several other states they can be quite lucrative and allow for frequent visits if the practitioner understands how to work within the system and do proper charting and reporting.

Personal Injury (PI)

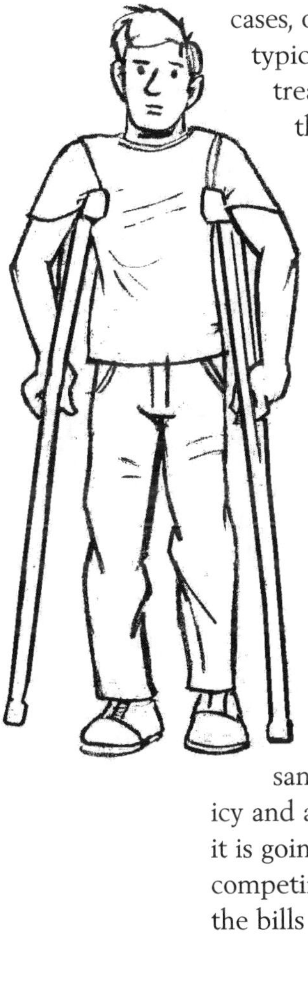

Personal injury (PI) cases are situations where a patient was involved in an accident that resulted in an injury caused by another individual or entity. The most common is a car accident though general liability cases, often called "slips and falls," are also possible. Attorneys are typically involved in these cases and the patient usually receives treatment immediately with the medical bills being paid when the court case is resolved. The patient and their attorney signs a "lien" outlining their promise to pay the medical bill out of the final settlement. PI cases require meticulous charting and reporting and often either a legal deposition or court appearance. They are also risky and may take several years to resolve. If the patient loses the case, the practitioner may not be paid. However, in the end, if the practitioner has chosen to treat a patient with a good case, they can usually receive a very lucrative payoff at the end: a large lump sum of cash based on the practitioner's full rates.

Med-pay, sometimes called personal injury protection (PIP), is part of a car insurance policy. This is like a mini fee-for-service insurance policy that pays for medical expenses associated with a car accident and avoids or postpones the necessity of a PI lien. A practitioner simply bills the car insurance company and gets reimbursed right away. There is one big wrinkle: they have a relatively low maximum for what they will pay out. And every practitioner is part of the same pool. In other words, if someone has a $5,000 med-pay policy and are seeing a medical doctor, chiropractor, and an acupuncturist, it is going to be maxed out pretty quickly. And the practitioners are competing on a first-come-first-served basis. The bottom line is to get the bills in quickly and check up on them frequently.

A patient may have an attorney with or without med-pay or med-pay with or without an attorney. It is always best to have the protection of an attorney, via a lien, whenever possible. If, however, the patient has a decent amount of med-pay and isn't seeing many providers, it may be okay that the patient doesn't also have an attorney. It's important to understand the nature of the case, assess its strength, viability, and ability to support and pay your bills.

Other types of insurance

There are some other types of insurance such as Medicare and TriCare that do not cover acupuncture. Medicare, the federal insurance program for the elderly, generally acts as fee-for-service insurance. While Medicare does not cover acupuncture, some Medicare supplemental insurance programs do. Medicaid is the federal insurance program for low-income individuals and families. While the federal program does not include acupuncture, it is administered by each state and some electively add coverage for acupuncture. MediCal, California's Medicaid program did, until recently, cover acupuncture at minimal levels. TriCare, the medical insurance for active duty military, does not cover acupuncture; though many VA programs do. Insurance for federal workers generally does not cover acupuncture. Is the theme apparent here? No federal insurance covers acupuncture. While there are bills in Congress to get it covered, they have gone nowhere for decades. A large hurdle for this coverage is the lack of acupuncture laws in all 50 states. The American Association of Acupuncture and Oriental Medicine is trying to get acupuncture federally covered.

Case Study

A prospective patient, Sally W., calls up to determine if her insurance policy can be used to pay for your services. She says she was in a car accident and has heard that acupuncture could help the healing process. What questions will you need to ask her? What other follow-up work might you need to do before you can decide to take her case? What type(s) of insurance may be involved?

1 Before Accepting Insurance

Before Accepting Insurance Checklist:

Whether or not you will be accepting insurance:

- Develop a fee schedule
- Create a HIPAA program
  — HIPAA Information handout for patients
- Determine technology needs (see Chapter 2)
- Get an NPI number
- Determine if you will be accepting insurance

If you are going to accept insurance:

- Start getting and filling out the paperwork for those insurance companies you wish to contract with
- Start figuring out the systems by thinking about work flow and starting to create any necessary forms
  — Probably, the most important form: Insurance Verification Form

There are many things to figure out before accepting insurance. Among these are the very basic question of should you accept insurance, setting up systems for keeping track of billing and other essentials, should you be in- or out-of-network, can you answer your patient's questions, and having all the paperwork and procedures ready to process claims. Most of these will be discussed throughout this book, but this chapter will discuss the first two questions.

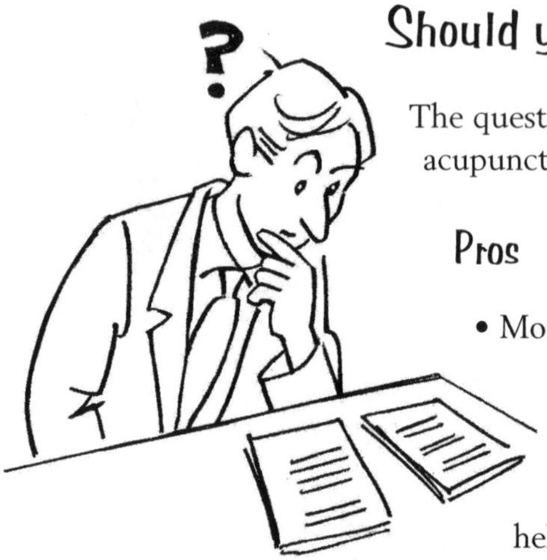

Should you accept insurance?

The question of accepting insurance is a big question for an acupuncturist. There are lots of pros and cons:

Pros

- More patients are able to afford your services. This leads to having more patients. Insurance allows patients who couldn't afford full rates to be able to get the healing they need. This is a helping profession and most acupuncturists enjoy helping others: more patients means more helping.
- There are lots of marketing benefits to accepting insurance. First, an acupuncturist doesn't need to say no or dodge the question when asked if they accept insurance. Second, if you are an in-network provider for a company, your name will be published in their directory which can drive patients to your practice, though this can sometimes take up to a year as they publish directories annually. Currently, most new providers are almost immediately available on the internet.
- A more lucrative practice. While some insurance companies pay less than most acupuncturists charge, others pay more. Workers' compensation, at least in California, pays very well. And, generally, more patients, even at less pay, means more money to the bottom line. The authors have never heard of relatively new, very successful practices, outside of elective practices such as reproductive medicine or facial rejuvenation, that do not accept insurance. We are sure they are out there (so please don't write letters), it is just easier to be really successful by accepting insurance.
- A more diverse practice. Having a mixture of patients including cash patients, insurance patients, workers' compensation patients, personal injury patients, and discount patients, means more diversity. More diversity means more ability to withstand shakeups in the regulatory environment or the economy. An example of this is when California, overnight, stopped paying workers' comp. We know many acupuncturists that went from

having very, very lucrative practices to bankruptcy in six months. By the same token, when the economy goes into a recession, many cash patients will not be able to afford acupuncture. But insurance patients can keep coming without much change in their pocketbook.
- Successfully taking insurance forces efficiencies. If one is not organized, it is difficult to take insurance and get paid on a regular basis. Accepting insurance means treating your patients more effectively both clinically and non-clinically.

Cons

- More paperwork. Potentially a lot more. Most of it, such as outcome assessments, should be done anyway, but some of it is insurance specific.
- Potentially less pay per patient. While many insurance companies do pay less than the average acupuncturist would charge, some pay more. Typically insurance pays $40-60 per patient visit. The other side is that you can see that patient more often (often insurance has limits to the number of visits, but generally not the frequency) and if you can see multiple patients in an hour, the hourly rate is not bad.
- You may not get paid, especially in the beginning when you need it the most. Billing insurance is a skill and it takes time to develop. While one is developing the skill, there will be mistakes, and while most can be recovered from, some cannot. That means losing money. For the most part, this lessens to almost nothing as experience is accumulated. Not to mention it is greatly lessened by reading a book such as this one.
- It adds one more thing to worry about and keep track of. Running a practice is already a very difficult endeavor, adding another thing to the pot may be daunting.
- Disorganized people will have a lot of trouble accepting and maintaining the systems necessary for insurance. But before the reader says, "Well, I am totally disorganized, therefore I can't do insurance," organization and building systems are skills not traits, genetic or otherwise. In other words, anyone can learn to do it.

But it does take the desire and effort. And some discipline in maintaining them.

- What is probably the biggest issue is ideological. We as acupuncturists tend to eschew the mainstream, otherwise we would be doctors or nurses. We like being out of the box. Insurance is as squarely "in the box" as it gets. To accept insurance means, to some, we buy into the "whole screwed up paradigm of medicine in this country." In the experience of the authors, this is probably the biggest hurdle to most acupuncturists accepting insurance.

There are obviously quite a few pros and cons to taking insurance and many more than are listed here. Many acupuncturists the authors have talked to have dabbled and then quickly retreated from accepting insurance. They will say things like, "I didn't get any more patients," "The paperwork was too much," "I never got paid," "It was too much of a hassle," or "It just wasn't worth it." All of these things are true. And many, very successful acupuncturists have worked out such issues. Most of these issues are resolved by waiting longer and spending more time learning the ropes. Successful acupuncturists interviewed for this book said that it takes, just like building a practice, at least a year or two until all of the benefits of accepting insurance started appearing and the downsides started becoming less frequent or disappeared. *So the take home lesson here is, if one does decide to accept insurance, it must be done for the long term. Do not dabble in it for six months and then give up.*

Another consideration is that in many parts of the country, we may be where chiropractors were 15 or 20 years ago and medical doctors were 20 or 30 years ago. At those times (and still), they were complaining and moaning about how insurance pays so little and their livelihoods will become much less lucrative. It was a time of transition from basically a cash basis or lucrative fee-for-service insurance practices to managed care practices. They kicked and screamed the entire time and yet now, most of these medical practitioners are part of the insurance game. The authors wonder if acupuncturists are at this stage, where we are being forced both from patients and insurance companies to play The Game, even though we don't want to. We may not have a huge choice. As a practitioner, are you going to be one of the bitter and resentful doctors bewailing the old days of easy money? Or will you realize this may be where our profession is, in all likelihood, inexorably headed and try to figure out the rules early and make not only the most of it, but actually thrive?

Using an insurance biller

The authors are often asked whether they should use an insurance biller if they decide to accept insurance. The answer is, as one would suspect, it depends. First off, the authors believe that it is imperative that practitioners do their own billing in the first six months to a year. This is because there are a lot of new things to learn and new ways of doing them, especially charting. The best way to accomplish this is to do all the billing by themselves. Usually, the amount of billing is not excessive and it is a powerful and natural learning curve. After this period, the decision rests on one question: how much insurance business are you generating? Most insurance billers charge on a percentage basis, so if you are doing enough business, it makes more sense to do it in-house and hire someone. If you are doing very little, it might be hard to find a competent biller. But if you are in the middle somewhere, a biller may be perfect. They may handle everything from verifications to follow-up on unpaid bills. The biggest caveat, however, is that you *must* get a biller with experience dealing with acupuncture billing as this is very different from other types of medical billing.

Case Study

Tom R. has just graduated from acupuncture college. He has been lucky and has only $45K in student loans, which he has deferred for one year. He has an offer to work out of a friend's chiropractic office, with possible referrals for both tuina and acupuncture patients. The chiropractor does accept certain types of insurance and is on a couple of managed care panels. Outline all the reasons why Tom may want to accept insurance and what types of insurance he should be familiar with billing. What are some of the concerns with accepting insurance?

Creating a system

In order to process insurance in an organized manner, a practitioner needs to have numerous systems in place to coordinate a patient's experience from start to finish. These include from when the patient first calls and insurance is verified to when the check is received from the insurance company. Systems are paramount to ensure that you have received all the necessary information to bill, get paid, and track your claims effectively. Not having these ready and operational will result in wasted time and, possibly, not getting paid.

The first order of business is to know with which insurance companies the practice is contracted. Deciding with whom to contract is very important and the application process is one of the first steps of accepting insurance. The process can take a while (months) so the earlier it is started, the sooner the practitioner will be able to start accepting insurance. Contact the provider relations/credentialing department for all matters relating to contracting, regardless of the insurance company. Below are the different types of insurance, with descriptions, to help decide with whom to contract. Generally before starting to contract with insurance companies, both individual practitioners and the overall practice must (legally) obtain a National Provider Identifier (NPI) number and possibly a tax identification number. This usually takes minutes over the internet and is discussed in further detail below.

In-network or out-of-network . . . what difference does it make?

Before sending out lots of contracts to various insurance companies, it is important to determine whether to be in- or out-of-network. Being an in-network provider means you are contracted with a particular insurance company. What does this actually mean? Sometimes it determines whether or not a practitioner is able to see a patient as stipulated by their individual type of coverage; whether they have in- or out-of-network benefits or only in-network.

Seeing an in-network provider typically means that a patient has better benefits and greatly reduced costs. Deductibles are sometimes waived when they see an in-network provider. Also, contracted providers are held to a fee schedule, as mandated by the contract, and therefore patient responsibilities can be reduced for this reason as well. It is almost always more beneficial for a patient to see an in-network physician as opposed to an out-of-network one.

There is one potentially big downside to being in-network. There are many laws that insurance companies must adhere to. But when a provider contracts with an insurance company the contract can limit these legal protections. For example, it is illegal for an insurance company to request or require a refund on a previously paid claim or claims. However, in almost every contract to be in-network, the provider agrees to allow refunds, if the insurance company incorrectly overpays.

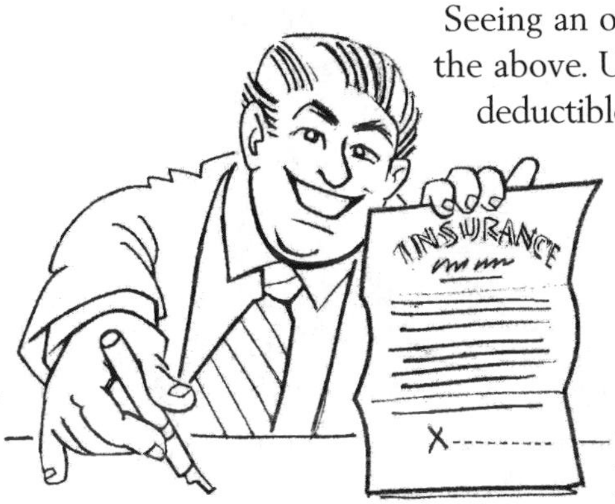

Seeing an out-of-network provider means the opposite of the above. Usually patient responsibilities are higher and deductibles apply, however, it gives the patient the option of seeing whichever provider they want. And practitioners may be paid more than if they were in-network.

In summary, there are several benefits and limitations to each. Being in-network gives the practitioner marketing benefits, but binds them to a contract which dictates what is paid and how it is paid, and what recourse and restrictions the practitioner must adhere to. Being out-of-network often means higher pay and fewer restrictions but has no marketing benefit. In addition, several big players, including American Specialty Health (ASH) and Kaiser Permanente, will not pay for out-of-network providers.

Health Maintenance Organizations (HMOs)

Health maintenance organizations are groups that providers can contract with, but need authorization for services prior to rendering treatment. Examples of these are American Specialty Health (ASH), Sharp Healthcare, and Kaiser Permanente. Being an ASH provider has its advantages and disadvantages… weigh them carefully before deciding to become a contracted provider.

The reasons to join ASH include being a provider for many other insurance companies as a result of your contract. They have a large patient database so there is the potential of getting a lot of patients through them. By being an ASH provider, you are able to see Kaiser Permanente patients, with a referral, since ASH manages Kaiser's authorizations and payments. Although ASH does require authorization for services, they allow you the first five visits without requiring authorization. The number of visits until authorization can increase over time. They have a website for all transmissions: authorization requests, eligibility verifications, and direct deposit information with a rapid turnaround for payments.

The disadvantages of being an ASH provider include needing authorization after the first five visits by creating and submitting a medical report, patients complain about filling out their paperwork, payment is a fraction of the typical cash rate for treatment, and many therapies are included in the reimbursement. Tracking the number of authorized visits can be troublesome. In addition, knowing when revised paperwork is needed may be difficult and can result in forfeiting the fee, because a provider is not allowed to charge the patient anything additional as stated in the contract. If you are unable to medically justify visits needed by the patient, as determined by ASH, the patient cannot be held financially responsible. By being a provider for ASH and any other insurance, contracts can sometimes cause additional fee reductions on workers comp and personal injury (PI) med-pay fees. For more specifics on different HMOs, see Appendix A.

General insurance

American Specialty Health (ASH) also oversees many general insurance companies. By being an ASH provider, you are automatically a provider for Blue Cross, Aetna, Cigna, and Health Net. *You must be contracted with ASH to be contracted with these carriers*. You cannot choose to be contracted with them and not ASH, it is all or nothing at this time. OptumHealth (formerly ACN) is the next largest network and they handle all contracting issues for United Healthcare, Pacificare, and Great West. Blue Shield is the only major payer who still handles their own contracting. These contractors may vary by state.

You will want to *verify* that these payers show you as a contracted provider in all their systems. Once you are a contracted provider, allow a month to go by and then either call the insurance companies to confirm that they show you as a provider or confirm when you are doing insurance verifications. Since they are updated by either ASH or OptumHealth, updates do not always happen as quickly as hoped. Verifying that these updates have actually occurred is very important. Also, make sure to check that the insurance websites have added you as a provider since this is how many prospective patients search for providers.

Workers' compensation (WC)

Joining medical provider networks (MPNs) for workers compensation (WC) is the next order of business, if you are in a state, such as California, that requires it. Once thought to be unnecessary, it has become increasingly important to be on these lists in order to treat WC patients. Most insurance carriers require you to belong to their MPN in order to treat their patients. The authors have actually received letters stating that an existing patient needs to stop treatment because the insurance company switched MPNs and we were not on the new MPN list. So, the more MPNs you are on the better to ensure the uninterrupted ability to treat in the event carriers change and to simply ensure you are available to as many patients as possible. Contact the major companies and see about joining their MPN. More on this in the workers compensation section.

Most WC companies are listed in the reference section of this book along with their contact information. For more information about joining an MPN, go to our website: www.acu-insurance.com, where you can click on links to take you directly to the MPN you are interested in joining. It also lists which MPN each insurance company is affiliated with.

Personal injury (PI) cases

There are no contracting requirements associated with personal injury (PI) cases. When someone comes in for a personal injury, you can treat them. You do *not* need a referral from a medical doctor or other healthcare provider to treat a patient under their PI case. There are many things to consider with regards to these types of cases, but they will be addressed in Appendix A and in chapter three. What you should know for purposes of this section is that there is a possibility of having your fees reduced slightly based on insurance contracts you may have, if your billing goes through a bill review process.

Contracting wrap-up

There should be a list of companies you are contracted with kept in a conspicuous place for staff members to reference when speaking with patients and insurance companies. Additionally, all of these insurance companies will need to have been updated with your National Provider Identifier (NPI) number (more on this later). This is how most general insurance companies are now identifying you as a healthcare practitioner. Few insurance companies have separate provider identification numbers.

Once a provider knows who they are contracted with or with whom they would like to join, the proper paperwork needs to be in place to handle their various forms requirements. Currently, of all the general insurance companies listed above, only ASH has special paperwork requirements. See the ASH section for more on the individual forms needed. Suffice it to say, the provider or their staff needs to know when a patient has ASH because they will have to complete specific forms at the onset of treatment and beyond. Having a system in place to handle ASH paperwork is necessary to be paid and remain a provider.

Closed panels

Closed panels are where, in a given location, the insurance company has determined they have enough providers of a certain specialty and will not add anyone else. In order to be reimbursed, a provider needs to be contracted with that insurance company. In other words, all providers are required to be in-network to be reimbursed **and** there is no way to be in-network at that moment in time.

First of all, this is perfectly legal and standard practice by many insurance companies. From their point of view, it means reduced administrative burdens and costs as well as having a select group of well-trained (in their system) practitioners. For providers on the panel, it is very advantageous as it means greatly reduced competition, many more patients, and more experience with that insurer. For providers outside of the panel, to put it in the vernacular, it sucks. That means you cannot see patients from that insurance company unless they are on a cash basis.

So how does one get on a closed panel? There are not any good rules on how to do this. Knowing someone on the inside helps. The best tip is probably to remain persistent. Turn in a request to be on the panel and respectfully follow-up on a regular basis, maybe monthly or quarterly. Eventually, when an opening does occur, you will be at the top of the list. Just do not be angry at the situation.

Health Insurance Portability and Accountability Act (HIPAA)

HIPAA is the Health Insurance Portability and Accountability Act. It was initially established primarily to protect electronically transmitted health information since online transmissions have skyrocketed in recent years and will eventually become mandatory. In the process of establishing confidentiality protocols, it broadened to more general office procedures. Many things that seem common sense became law such as:

- Do not discuss patient conditions where other people could potentially hear you (this applies to office staff as well as practitioners).
- Do not disclose personal information (social security numbers, dates of birth, etc.) such that non-staff can hear you.
- Turn computer monitors away from non-staff viewing.
- Do not keep any healthcare records in plain view so they could be easily viewed by mistake.

- Patient sign-in sheets *are* acceptable although they were initially thought to be banned as well.
- Patient files that are stored in file pockets on patient room doors should face inward, not outward, so patient names are not readable.

Verifying the legitimacy of patient inquiries is also necessary. Not releasing information to anyone other than the patient, unless you have authorization in writing from the patient, is of huge importance. This is done in the same way that insurance companies do to us: they ask for verifying information such as date of birth (DOB) and policy and/or social security numbers prior to relinquishing information regarding a patient. You must have express written consent to send records on a patient to anyone other than the patient unless they have been subpoenaed. HIPAA violations are handled by the office of civil rights and with an office in each major city in the United States, complaints made regarding HIPAA are readily investigated. Fines begin at $500. The point: it is easy for a patient to file a complaint and relatively easy for bureaucrats to follow up on it and so every practice must have a HIPAA system in place.

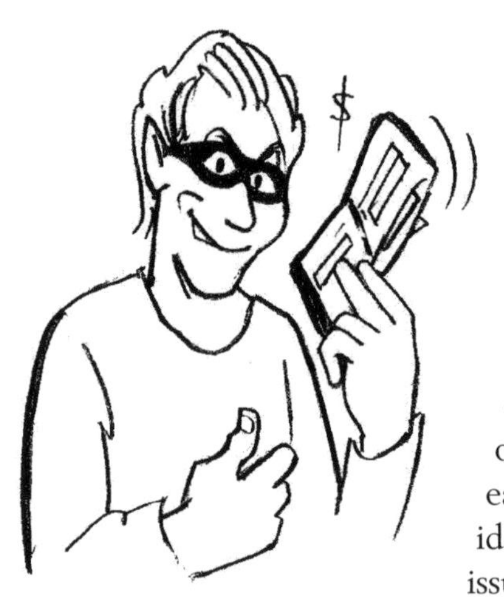

Identity theft

Along the same lines as HIPAA and with an increased threat of identify theft due to enhanced computer technology, there are now policies that your office should follow regarding prevention of identity theft. Some of these are already commonly used in retail establishments, but are being brought to even small office environments to curb the problem. Since each office already gets a copy of each patient's valid identification (ID) (driver's license, military- or state-issued ID) for their charts, each practice should be well on their way to compliance. The difference is one should examine this documentation relative to their payment method. First, does the information stated on their intake forms match their ID (address, DOB, picture, signature)? If not, inquire for clarification and act or notate accordingly. If the patient gives you a health insurance card, does the name match that on the ID? If they pay with a check or credit card, do the names on them match the ID? Ongoing awareness of these practices will help minimize the risk of identify theft happening at your practice. Just as one is supposed to hold periodic HIPAA awareness meetings, a similar discussion about prevention of identity theft should occur and be documented. Though recent (Dec. 2010) law clarified that medical professionals do not fall under the Federal Trade Commission's regulation (called the "Red Flags Rule") requiring an identity theft policy, it is still a good business practice to do so.

Electronic billing

Many claims can be submitted using online access. Some individual insurance companies allow you to enter claims directly on their websites, although this can require time-consuming data entry. If you are manually completing claims anyway, then this is a potential method you might want to use to get paid faster. You would have to inquire with each insurance company, via their provider relations department, how to use each individual site. If you have a Practice Management System (PMS) that automatically generates claims for you, then a better electronic method is to subscribe to a clearinghouse. Using this method, your claims are automatically downloaded (instead of printed) to a clearinghouse who filters your claims for you and distributes them to the various insurance companies. One author uses Emdeon by WebMD a popular clearinghouse but others are available and could be found via a web search. This is a much more efficient system for claims submission and gets your claims paid faster, usually within about two weeks. If one is an ASH provider, claims should always be submitted via their website since there are incentives for completing them online. Once direct deposit is initiated, online submission of claims usually means payments are received within 7-10 days.

You will not always be able to submit claims electronically; there are still many smaller insurance companies that do not accept electronic claims and so they will have to be printed and mailed.

National Provider Identifier (NPI)

It used to be that all you needed to bill, in terms of an identification number, was your Tax Identification Number (TIN). A TIN is either a social security number or an Employer Identification Number (EIN), if there are employees. This is no longer the case. Recently mandated, all healthcare providers who transmit information electronically, must bill with an NPI (National Provider Identifier) number. Obtaining an NPI is very simple. Log on to: https://nppes.cms.hhs.gov, click the 'Apply online for an NPI' and complete the necessary questions. You will be issued an NPI within 48 hours. You will also need to obtain an NPI for the clinic or group. Which number you bill with (individual or group) is determined by how the individual insurance company recognizes you, the provider. You will also need to decide if you need an EIN or if you will use your social security number for tax purposes. If you have any employees, you will need an EIN. If you are a single practitioner with a sole proprietorship and no employees, you can use your social security number. For privacy reasons, so that your social security number isn't distributed regularly and/or to be prepared for the future when you hire an employee, you may want to get an EIN. Since the process of changing information after the fact (TIN, addresses, etc.) can be problematic with insurance companies, it is least painful to establish oneself from the get go.

Developing a fee schedule

A fee schedule is a legal requirement for a medical practice. Let's rephrase this, if a practitioner does not have a fee schedule or is not consistent with an existing one, they are open to allegations of fraud and will have no defense against them. And there have been acupuncturists who have been *convicted* of fraud, so this is a real worry.

A fee schedule should include every service your practice bills for as well as any products sold. A sample fee schedule can be found on pages 25–26 below and at our website at www.acu-insurance.com.

This book does not specifically go into how much to charge for any of the procedures discussed. There are several reasons for this. In a free, capitalist society, the biggest no-no is to have monopolistic powers (unless granted by the government). To have specific amounts in this book would be legally considered to be collusion and therefore tantamount to creating a monopoly and illegal. Having said that, there are guidelines for reimbursement amounts. These are called the Resource Based Relative Value Scale (RBRVS).

Resource Based Relative Value Scale (RBRVS)

The RBRVS is a set of guidelines developed by the AMA and supplemented by the Centers for Medicare and Medicaid Services (CMS). These guidelines determine the baseline for how much Medicare will pay medical providers for certain services and equipment. There are three variables:

Relative Value Units (RVUs): These units are a number representing the cost for a given procedure or service. There are three components of these costs: physician's work, practice expense, and malpractice costs. For example, the RVU for an acupuncture treatment (CPT code 97810; more on CPT codes later in the book) is .95.

Geographic Practice Cost Index (GPCI): This is a number that varies according to where the physician is located and takes into account the fact that it may be more expensive in some locations than others. For example, Los Angeles' GPCI is higher than that of Arkansas'. The problem is that there is a separate GPCI for each of the three components that make up the RVU (physician's work, practice expense, and malpractice) and therefore this gets very complicated very quickly. The bottom line is geography influences how much each service is reimbursed under Medicare.

Conversion Factor (CF): This is how much each RVU is worth in terms of dollars. As of March, 2011, the CF is $33.9764. Please note, however, that this number changes on a regular basis. To find the most current cost factor check our website or the Centers for Medicare and Medicaid Services (CMS)."

Each of these variables, for commonly used CPTs, can be found either at our website, www.acu-insurance.com, or the AMA's (www.ama-assn.org) or CMS's (www.cms.hhs.gov) websites.

In its simplest—and not entirely accurate—form, the amount reimbursed is equivalent to multiplying each of these variables together. If we don't consider the GPCI, this means that acupuncture should be reimbursed by Medicare at .95 x 33.9764 which equals $32.28. This of course isn't accurate. First, Medicare does not pay for acupuncture. Second, this does not take into account where the service is performed. But this can be used as a guideline. Generally the Medicare reimbursement is about the lowest an insurance company will pay. Your fees should probably be based on this number but be a multiple of it. In one of the authors' practice, the fee schedule is based on over 2 times this figure. Using a multiple of Medicare reimbursement is probably the easiest, most accurate, and most defensible way to develop a fee schedule. It is also one of the rarest ways in our profession.

Fee schedule

Most acupuncturists develop their fees by figuring out how much they want to charge for a visit and including everything they do in that fee. For example, an acupuncturist may charge $60 (this number is not based on anything nor is it a suggestion of any kind) for a visit and provide acupuncture, heat packs on the back, a heat lamp on the feet, and massage with liniment for a few minutes after the acupuncture. This will not work for insurance billing (see form below).

Insurance billing requires a separate code (Current Procedural Terminology [CPT] codes, described in Chapter 5 on charting) for each procedure or service performed. Each of the services described in the previous paragraph has a separate code. And each is individually reimbursable. This has pros and cons. It may mean that you can get

Fee Schedule

Fees listed below are for illustration purposes only and should not be construed as suggestive or illustrative of actual fees

CPT	Description	Fee	20% Cash (in CA) or Time of Service Discount
97810 (97800 WC*)	Acupuncture	$19.14	$15.31
	Initial 15 mins		
97811	Acupuncture	$14.78	$11.82
	Additional 15 mins		
97813 (97801 WC*)	Electroacupuncture	$20.46	$16.37
	Initial 15 mins		
97814	Electroacupuncture	$16.67	$13.34
	Additional 15 mins		
E&M New Patient			
99201	Problem-Focused	$18.38	$14.70
99202	Expanded	$32.59	$26.07
99203	Detailed	$48.51	$38.81
99204	Moderate Complex	$68.59	$54.88
99205	Highly Complex	$87.16	$69.73
Established Patient			
99211	Minimal	$10.80	$ 8.64
99212	Problem-Focused	$19.33	$15.46
99213	Expanded	$26.34	$21.07
99214	Moderate Complex	$41.31	$33.05
99215	Highly Complex	$60.07	$48.05
Consultations			
99241	Problem-Focused	$25.20	$20.16
99242	Expanded	$46.05	$36.84
99243	Detailed	$61.39	$49.12
99244	Moderate Complex	$86.60	$69.28
99245	Highly Complex	$111.99	$89.59

WC* indicates codes that the California Workers' Compensation system currently uses, however at the time of writing this, it looks as though this is going to change in the near future.

continued on next page . . .

Fee Schedule (continued)

CPT	Description	Fee	20% Cash (in CA) or Time of Service Discount
Procedures			
97110	Therapeutic procedure 15 mins, develop strength, endurance, ROM, flexibility	$14.02	$11.22
97112	Neuromuscular re-education movement, balance, coord., posture	$14.59	$11.67
97124	Massage	$11.18	$8.94
97140	Manual therapy techniques mobilization, manipulation, lymphatic drainage, traction 15 mins	$13.07	$10.46
Modalities			
97010	Hot/cold packs	$2.27	$1.82
97012	Traction mechanical	$7.39	$5.91
97014	E-stim unattended	$7.20	$5.76
97032	Application of modality to one or more areas E-stim (manual) each 15 mins	$7.96	$6.37
Tests & Measurements			
97750	Physical performance test for measurement (e.g. musculoskeletal, functional capacity) w/written report each 15 mins	$14.97	$11.98
Supplies			
A4215	Needles	$ 1.50	$ 1.50
99049	Missed appointments communication purposes only	???	???

Assumptions: Fees are based on RVU values multiplied by a cost factor of 33.9764 and an internal multiplier of .5. WC* indicates codes that the California Workers Compensation system currently uses, however at the time of writing this, it looks as though this is going to change in the near future.

more money than the $60 by listing each service separately. Of course, insurance may not pay an acupuncturist for each of these services. Or insurance companies may deny some of them but not all of them, meaning more paperwork hassles. But many will pay for each and every one. In California's workers compensation system, the reimbursement for the treatment described in the previous paragraph would be around $117. Anyway you look at it, improper coding, including packaged services, is unethical, possibly illegal, and can have ramifications.

A proper fee schedule will have individual codes and how much is charged for each of these codes. Charting should include individual services and their corresponding charges. What the charges are for each code is completely up to the individual practitioner. While these charges can be influenced by competition, geographic location, and other business factors, there should not be any hint of collusion involved. Collusion is where several competitors sit down together and say they want to charge a patient (or customer) the same thing and artificially inflate consumer cost. In other words, it is okay to call around and see what other acupuncturists are charging in your area and then decide how much you want to charge. But it is illegal to invite everyone to pizza and decide that you are all going to charge $75 per acupuncture treatment. For this reason, the associations in our profession cannot answer any questions or research how much acupuncturists charge their patients. A commonly used reference for charges might be a variation of the California Workers Comp fee schedule.

Whether or not a provider bills insurance, they should have a fee schedule and stick by it. Legally, a patient may request a copy of the fee schedule and the provider must supply it. Not having one and using it consistently can leave the door open to charges of fraud if anything goes wrong with billing.

Discounts

It is legal and probably desirable to offer discounts to certain individuals, so long as they are clearly determined in your fee schedule. Generally the base fee, and the most expensive, is what you plan to charge insurance. This doesn't mean you will get this with each company, but you still bill the same. For example, if your fee for an acupuncture treatment is $100, but you know XYZ insurance company will only reimburse you $50, you still bill the full $100. Always. You will have to write off the $50 not received through accounting procedures, but everything will be done legally. What is illegal is charging XYZ company $50 while charging ABC company $100.

So what kind of discounts should be offered? First, the insurance rate should be a good deal higher than what is reimbursed. This is because some insurance companies will pay higher than others and a practitioner doesn't want to leave money on the table. So that means charging $100 or $150 for an acupuncture treatment is not unreasonable. There are a couple situations where you can be reimbursed at these levels.

But the average patient isn't going to pay $150 once or twice a week for acupuncture. So the first and most important discount is for patients who don't have insurance. There are two ways to provide this discount.

California discounts. In California, the law is very generous and allows a separate "noninsured" discounted fee and a "cash" fee. These fees can be any value you would like and you may offer one or both. There can be an economic hardship fee on a sliding scale, so long as that scale is structured, predetermined, and consistently applied. It may look a little suspicious if the noninsured fee is dramatically different than the insured fee.

Discounts for the rest of the country. In most of the rest of the country, it is illegal to bill insurance more than an uninsured patient. There is a way around this though. You can have a Time Of Service (TOS) discount. This is a discount that is given only if the bill is paid at the same time as (or before) the service is performed. Technically, if an insurance company could pay in advance or on the day of the treatment, they would be eligible for this discount. But because that never happens, it becomes a discount for uninsured or cash patients. These TOS discounts should be clearly delineated in your fee schedule.

As a note of caution, insurance law is different in individual states and a practitioner should always be well versed in the insurance laws of their state, in addition to federal insurance laws.

Other discounts. In the fee schedule, you can delineate discounts for any "class" you would like. You might want to provide discounts for senior citizens, students, military personnel, friends, your sewing or soccer buddies, or any other group of patients. The trick here is to make sure they are applied consistently. In other words, a definition of who qualifies for the discount is needed and then everyone who qualifies actually receives the discount every time.

Offering discounts to "protected classes" are considered discriminatory and highly illegal. These protected classes are anything based upon race, gender, religion, and disability. The reason for this is by giving a discount to one of these classes you are excluding the rest within that class. For example, if you want to give a discount to Wiccans and Jews, you are excluding Christians and Muslims from that discount and therefore discriminating on the basis of religion, which is illegal under both state and federal law (Healy, 2008).

Sliding scale discounts are possible in many states. In general, they are illegal unless the state has a specific legal exemption allowing them. In those states where it is legal, it does not mean you can charge whatever you want to whomever you want. You need to establish a firm scale, based on income levels and you need to have patient documentation supporting those incomes in order to give them the discount (Healy, 2008).

What to tell patients

After so many practitioners charge a straight fee, even though this does not serve for insurance purposes, it is hard to try to explain that you charge according to the services you perform. A way around this is to use the following script when a potential patient asks how much it costs:

"Just like a doctor, we don't know what we are going to need to do or how much it is going to cost until we see you. A typical initial visit will cost between $xxx and $xxx, usually on the lower end, and subsequent visits usually run from $xxx-$xxx, again usually on the lower end of this range. If you would like, we will be happy to provide you with a copy of our fee schedule."

Most patients readily accept this explanation of charges and it is in complete alignment with how most medical professionals bill their patients.

Summary

In summary, to run a practice legally and to minimize the chances of being prosecuted for insurance fraud, a practitioner needs to develop a fee schedule that outlines all the fees and discounts offered. All procedures offered by the practitioner should be on the schedule. Please see the section on CPT codes in Chapter 5 for potential codes to include.

Sam Collins (Oct., 2008), an expert in insurance billing, states four criteria for an appropriate fee schedule. A fee schedule should be reasonable, defensible, consistent, and publicized. Reasonable is justified by looking at other acupuncturists in your area and top reimbursement rates, be they insurance or workers compensation. By using RBRVS as a basis of your fee schedule, it is defensible. You as a practitioner and your staff need to apply it consistently. And it should be public, either upon request or as part of the patient's initial paperwork.

Fee schedules should be reassessed on an annual basis by looking at changing economics and medical reimbursement rates. A practitioner can change the fee schedule as necessary, though annually is most appropriate. It is good business practice to warn patients several months **in advance of any fee increase.**

Case Study

Where Kim S. went to school, there was one price for a treatment and a patient may have received acupuncture, a short massage, an herbal recommendation, and maybe have a heat lamp placed over his or her feet. As Kim tries to determine what to charge in her new practice, she calls local acupuncturists who tell her a new patient is charged X while returning patients are charged Y. Is this legal? Is it ethical? Does Kim need to develop a fee schedule?

Technology in the Acupuncturist's Office

2

Chapter 2 Checklist:

- Choosing appropriate hardware
- Which operating system works best for your office needs?
- Desktop or laptop or tablet?
- Software needs in a clinic that bills insurance

Technology plays an important role in the modern acupuncturist's office. Of course technology encompasses everything from your telephone system to an electrical stimulation machine. This section, however, will concentrate on computers, including hardware, software, and peripherals. If an acupuncturist is going to accept insurance, it is almost mandatory to have an appropriate computer system with access to the internet. While it might be possible to do an exclusively paper-oriented insurance business, there would be no access to online verification, one would not be able to properly bill American Specialty Health (ASH), and eventually, Medicare and the rest of the insurance companies will demand online submissions only. In other words, the future looks bleak for paper insurance submissions. Besides, once learned, electronic submissions are much easier than paper. Cheaper too.

Hardware

The first major decision to make in regards to hardware is to determine the operating system. Operating systems are the software that makes the hardware work. Deciding on an operating system often drives the hardware decision. There are three major operating systems currently: Windows, Mac OS, and Linux. Each of these may have different flavors (such as Windows XP, Vista, or 7, or in the case of Linux, multiple "distros" or distributions). One of the authors was a computer consultant for eight years (that is how he helped pay for Oriental medical school), and his advice in regards to hardware decisions was to find the software you want to run, then buy the hardware that will run it for the next 3-5 years. Given this advice, the next sections discuss each of the operating systems.

Operating systems

Windows

Windows is by far the most common operating system on computers with a market share hovering somewhere near the 90% mark. There are several pros and cons to this system. Almost all software will run on Windows. While it is almost exclusively the target of malware (malicious software such as viruses and spyware), a con, it is also patched more quickly than any of the other operating systems, a pro. Almost every peripheral will run on a Windows system. The most current version of Windows as we go to press is Windows 7. It has been received with nearly universally good reviews and appears to be the best version yet. In general, almost all of the software that one would like to run in an acupuncturist's office not only will run on Windows, it must run on Windows. For business, Windows is almost the only real choice for a computer system. And before the Mac attack begins, please read the next section.

Mac OS

Macintosh OS, currently, as this is written, on version Mac OS X Snow Leopard, is an incredibly powerful operating system using Macintosh hardware built exclusively by Apple. Pros for this operating system include ease of use, very powerful graphics and video software, minimal malware incidents, and a very happy and tight cadre of fellow users. Cons include a very happy and tight cadre of fellow users (some call them fanatics), expense, as the hardware tends to run several hundred dollars more than comparable Windows hardware, fewer peripheral choices, and in the business world, fewer people/ employees familiar with Mac OS. The biggest con, however, is software compatibility, and, despite a few exceptions, all major business and medical software works exclusively with the Windows operating system. However, since Apple went to Intel CPU chips several years ago, the systems now include the ability to run Windows in addition to Mac OS. This sounds ideal at first glance until one realizes it is not an easy switch. It means learning two operating systems, switching between them can be quite time-consuming, and Windows may run slower and not be completely the same as on a dedicated Windows system, though these last two issues are probably not relevant to business and medical software as neither are too taxing on the hardware. The bottom line is: the Apple Macintosh is a great system, especially if the user is familiar with or wants to use graphic arts programs, but it is not a primary business system. In addition, as we will explore below, there are some interesting hardware options not available from Apple.

Linux

Linux is an open-source (meaning it is created and maintained by volunteers and is essentially free) version of an old operating system, Unix —which, as an aside, is what Mac OS X is based on. It is a powerful system that has little hardware overhead, meaning it can run faster than other operating systems on cheaper hardware. Unfortunately, it is the most difficult of these systems to learn, use, and maintain. While almost all of the software is free, it is difficult to find top-notch medical software and the variety of software is limited. In business, Linux is usually relegated to the role of web server where it has a dominant market share. Rarely, is it used as a primary operating system, especially in a medical office.

Hardware platforms

Hardware comes in a variety of form factors including desktop, laptop, tablet, and handheld. In general, desktops are the least expensive and most powerful form factor, though laptops are rapidly closing these gaps. Desktops generally are not portable, though a new breed of small form factors may be portable. These include the Apple Mini and the Dell Studio. Laptops are portable and go from the very small netbooks to the large desktop replacements. In between these two extremes, lie the ultraportable, value, and business laptops. While netbooks probably aren't powerful enough to run an acupuncturist's office alone, any of the other types of laptops can be and which to choose comes down to personal preference.

Laptops can also flow into another category of computer: the Tablet PC. These are computers with screens you can write on and can convert handwriting to text. These can be very useful in the medical office as it is possible to write your chart notes directly on the screen. These PCs come in two varieties: convertible and slate. Convertible tablet PCs look and act like ordinary laptops but the screen can rotate and fold flat to write on. These have all the advantages of being both a laptop and Tablet PC though they are heavier than the slate. They are built by Lenovo (formerly IBM), Fujitsu, Gateway, Hewlett Packard, and Dell among others. Slate Tablet PCs are exclusively a big screen and do not have an attached keyboard (but you can add one). They are generally lighter than the convertible but not as convenient. The main company building these is Motion Computing. Another advantage of the Tablet PCs, besides writing chart notes, is when presenting something from a program such as PowerPoint, one can draw directly on the presentation making it much more exciting and interactive.

The final form factor is the handheld device. These include operating systems such as iPhone, Windows Mobile, Symbian, Android, PalmOS, (now called WebOS), and Blackberry. None of these could run a practice, but they can be very useful for reference and portable scheduling. Any of these can do basic scheduling, and most have medical and Oriental medical reference software available. The iPhone has some absolutely gorgeous reference programs. PalmOS has quite a few programs as well, though they tend to be a little less graphic than other types of handhelds. Many of these programs have free trial periods and the authors recommend thoroughly exploring a program before purchasing. For more information and links on these programs check out our website at www.acu-insurance.com.

The iPad and Android-based tablets are rapidly becoming very popular though are not useful (yet) for running a practice. They can, however, be very helpful in many ways including searching for references and research and for educating patients.

The bottom line in hardware is to look at your software needs and buy hardware that will run them. In general, for basic medical office functionality, buying on the low end of the spectrum probably will be more than adequate.

Software

Many different kinds of software are necessary to run a successful practice and to bill insurance. These include office programs, accounting software, practice management systems (PMS), and possibly electronic medical record (EMR) or electronic healthcare record (EHR) software and graphics software for creating flyers and forms. In addition, some basic software that should be on any system include virus and anti-malware programs. And many of these programs need to be assessed for HIPAA concerns.

Before talking about software, a general warning needs to be said. While as a student or not, an individual may have a few copied programs on their computer. While this is completely illegal and the authors certainly do not condone it, the chances of being caught and punished is practically zero unless one is involved in distributing them. This is not the case for businesses. In business, each computer must have its own copy of the software or a software license. Businesses are often caught and the penalties are severe with a maximum fine of $150,000 *per copied program* with the added possibility of jail time if there is "willful piracy" (Software & Information Industry Association, 2009). Businesses do get caught and they are fully prosecuted. So please do not use copied software in your business, the risk is very real and very large. In conjunction with this, a lot of "free" programs are only free for a consumer. But a company may need to pay for it, so please read the license agreement for any "free" software used in your business.

Office programs

General office programs are necessary for the smooth operation of a practice. Necessary office programs include a word processor, a spreadsheet, and an email program often coupled with a scheduling and contact list program. In addition, presentation software can be very useful and is usually included in an office software package. Microsoft Office is the grand daddy of the office packages. It is very widely used, is the standard for compatibility, and is very (some people say too) powerful, which may make it more difficult to learn. The biggest drawback is the expense, as it can be quite costly, especially if there are multiple computers in the office. OpenOffice is a free open-source alternative that is almost as powerful as Microsoft Office, but does tend to have a few glitches in compatibility. Star Office is another alternative. The internet offers some very viable if not as strong alternatives such as GoogleDocs or Zoho Office. These are particularly useful when several people need to collaborate on the same document.

Desktop publishing or other graphics software are sometimes included in these packages and can be a great help in creating flyers and forms for the office. The only caveat is, you generally need some level of expertise or the willingness to learn these programs in order for them to be useful.

Accounting software

Accounting software may be necessary to run a business. If you are keeping track of your own finances then you need to get some software. The most popular accounting package is QuickBooks by Intuit. QuickBooks Simple Start is a limited free version. Peachtree accounting is also very popular. The authors suggest getting a bookkeeper because they will be cheaper in the long run as the practitioner should be spending his/her time treating patients and marketing themselves. If you do need to buy accounting software, talk to your certified public accountant (CPA) to determine what is compatible with their systems.

Practice Management Software/Systems (PMS)

Practice management software (PMS) assist all the front office functions of a medical practice. These include scheduling, billing, and other administrative issues. There are no clear-cut leaders in this software category, but some things to look for include the financial stability of the company, depth of features, its form factor (whether it is server based, on the web, or on individual computers), ease of use, and costs including necessary hardware, maintenance, and training. One author really likes Eclipse software (www.galactek.com) which is very powerful but can be expensive (though it can be leased for a reasonable amount). The other author likes www.officeally.com, which is free for its PMS functions, but considerably less powerful and slower.

Electronic healthcare record (EHR) software

Electronic healthcare records (EHR) is the same thing as electronic charting and is also called electronic medical recordkeeping (EMR). The practitioner produces his/her charts on their computer eliminating or minimizing paper charting (some of the initial paperwork may still be paper). Advantages of this include greatly reduced costs in supplies and storage, filing of paperwork, and ease of accessibility. Disadvantages include the cost, dealing with the change in workflow, and training. Another question mark is about security. Since most of us who have used computers have experienced at least one catastrophic failure and loss of data, it is felt that EHRs may be less safe than paper. However, if done properly with off-site backups, studies have shown paper records are much more susceptible to mishaps including floods, fires, and earthquakes. So, as long as a reputable company is used, EHRs are much safer than paper. Another consideration when thinking about EHR software is that Medicare, and subsequently other insurance companies, have stated their intention to go exclusively to electronic submission of claims (more of a PMS and front office function) with only electronic records being accepted to support claims (this is where EHRs come in). This has been slated to begin in the next few years, but the deadlines have been consistently pushed back for decades. President Obama's revamping of the healthcare system includes EHRs. In deciding which EHR program to use, practitioners should take into account cost, ease of use, the stability of the software publishing company, and the extensive use of standards so that the information can be used within the healthcare system.

Software summary

In reality, software will probably be a considerably bigger expense than hardware and time should be spent in determining the office's needs and which software will accomplish those needs. Remember, the cost of software is not just about buying the appropriate package. Installation and training costs must also be figured in. And buying the wrong package can be very expensive directly and indirectly. As a rule, one should not buy software without thoroughly assessing its demo software. If a demo is not available, pass on the software.

3 Before a Patient Arrives

Before a Patient Arrives Checklist:

- Find out if the patient has insurance
- If so, get their insurance information using an insurance verification form
  - — Contact the insurance company and verify benefits
  - — Inform the patient of their benefits
- If the patient is a workers' compensation patient
  - — Patient needs to have a prescription and authorization for acupuncture
- If the patient is a personal injury case
  - — Patient needs to bring their auto insurance information, health insurance for verification, attorney information (if applicable) and accident report, if they have it.

Benefits

Benefits are what an insured individual receives from the insurance company, according to their policy, for services rendered. Some policies cover acupuncture and others do not. The *most* important step in accepting insurance is finding out what the benefits cover. There are several steps and lots of jargon to learn in order to accomplish this. This process is called verification of benefits. This chapter will also discuss how to deal with both an insurance company who is not being forthright with information and an individual who has been denied.

Patient calls to schedule appointment

After scheduling an appointment, ask if they have insurance or if the appointment will be related to workers compensation or an auto or other type of accident. If the visit will be due to a workers compensation or accident, the patient needs to know what information to bring to their appointment. If this doesn't happen, the authors *highly* recommend that it be the first question on your patient intake form: "Is this a work related injury or auto accident?" If so, *stop* and inform the front desk to give your patient the correct paperwork. The front desk staff should also reiterate this question before handing new patients their paperwork. If they have insurance, ask to verify it ahead of time. This will work out in some but not all cases. The below questions apply to pre-verification of benefits and are based on the case type:

Insurance

Ask if 1) the patient can fax or email a copy of their insurance card to the office, preferably enlarged, and make sure the toll free customer service phone number and their date of birth (DOB) is written on the fax as well *or* 2) ask them to read the identification number, their name, date of birth, and the customer service number and the office staff would be glad to check. Depending on your conversation, staff may want to call the patient back *prior* to their appointment to inform them of their benefits or it might be fine to let them know their benefits when they come in for their appointment. It is always best to try and verify benefits *prior* to the appointment in case you do not have the time to call while the patient is there (if the office gets busy), or there may be difficulty getting through to the insurance company for various reasons. If there is no verification of benefits, the office will not know if the patient has benefits. This may impair your office from scheduling further appointments or mean that your office does not know how to correctly charge the patient.

Workers' compensation

A workers' comp patient needs to have a prescription and an authorization to receive acupuncture before services are rendered. This should happen before making an initial appointment.

If the patient is a workers' comp case, make sure they provide their adjusters information along with the prescription for acupuncture from their primary treating physician. Authorization may not have been obtained yet, in which case you will need to get this prior to initiating a course of treatment. For more on the work comp authorization process, see the section on workers' compensation in Appendix A.

Personal injury (PI)

The patient should bring their auto insurance as well as health insurance information to the appointment. If they have an attorney, they should bring this information as well. If they have any other information pertinent to the case, they should bring it as well (accident report, letters from their auto insurance, medical records from another medical provider, etc.). Please remember that a practitioner does not need to accept a PI patient. If the case does not look good, do not take it.

Verifying benefits

All health insurance verifications begin with a phone call to the insurance company. There is a toll free customer service number on the patient's insurance card which is the start of verification. Every practice should develop proper forms to fill out during the verification of benefits. Certain information about the patient is necessary to verify benefits. This should be included on the insurance verification form prior to the call (see below). Verification forms should also be made for workers comp and personal injury/med-pay cases since each requires slightly different information. The information necessary for each verification type is discussed below.

A note about verification via the internet: as of this date, the only insurance company that you can rely on to offer complete on-line benefit information is American Specialty Health (ASH). It is best when verifying an ASH patient to use their on-line system since it is very clear and can be printed and put into the patient's file. On the other hand, all other insurance companies' on-line benefit information is, in the authors' opinions, insufficient to conclusively derive the patient's acupuncture benefits. Most companies have the major medical information and, although many are including acupuncture benefits, there are questions unanswered via their on-line benefits. These include whether there is a deductible, how much has been met, how many visits have been used out of their benefits thus far, etc. Unfortunately, it is still better to call for benefits to all insurance companies except ASH. For personal injury and workers compensation cases, phone calls are *always* required to verify benefits and eligibility.

Health insurance verification form—this form should include the date, patient's name, date of birth, insurance company name and identification number, as well as your National Provider Identifier (NPI) and Tax I.D. number (TIN) for easy reference. It should address the following: are there acupuncture benefits? If so, are they in- or out-of-network benefits? If a provider is not sure about their network affiliation, ask them to check your NPI/TIN.

Is there a deductible, if so, how much and how much has been met? Does their plan go by calendar year or fiscal year (usually starting in July)? How many visits does the patient have per year, have any been used? Or is there a dollar limit per year, if so, has any been used? Is there a set copay or is it a coinsurance? A copay is a set dollar amount that the patient will owe per visit versus the coinsurance that is a percent of the allowable amount that is the patient's responsibility per visit. For example, when they quote you benefits of 80%, this automatically means that the patient's coinsurance is the other 20% and of course the patient has no copay since they have coinsurance; it's a one or the other scenario. On the other hand, the patient's coverage may cover 100% with a copay of $10; this means that the patient's only financial responsibility for the visit is $10. If the patient has no coverage, ask if there are any discount programs. It is good practice to ask what the timeframe for claim submissions is and start to keep a list for future reference. One needs to get or confirm the claims submission address and ask if there are any special submission requirements. Always ask and document who the representative was, the date, and a reference number for the call. The person in your office who completed the form should also initial it. A sample of this form can be found on page 183 or visit our website to download a sample. Of note: if you are an out-of-network provider, you are not required to accept the insurance-allowed amounts. You can bill patients the difference between what you billed and what was paid by insurance.

Case Study

Sally F. called to schedule an appointment with Rick but wanted to know if her insurance covered acupuncture first. After offering to call and verify the coverage for her, the insurance informed our office that Rick was not showing as a provider and so the service would not be covered. Although he should have shown up as a contracted provider, there was an issue that was able to be remedied shortly thereafter. Had Rick treated the patient when scheduled, the visit would not have been covered forcing the patient to unexpectedly pay out-of-pocket, in-full. The patient was re-scheduled with Rick two weeks later after the contracting issue was resolved. Always reconfirm the practitioner's providership when verifying insurance.

The workers' compensation verification form should include the claim number, date of injury, insurance company name and address for claims, the adjuster's name, phone and fax numbers along with the utilization reviewer's (UR) phone and fax numbers. Ensuring the claim is open and active should be verified as well. If there is an attorney on the case, you should get their information as well. Also ask if they require submission of anything with the claim (i.e., chart notes, authorization, etc.). See sample on next page.

Personal injury (PI)/med-pay verification forms include much of the same information as workers compensation forms. Since there is an adjuster assigned to these types of claims as well, the adjuster's information should be recorded along with the claim number and date of injury. The patient's auto insurance company's name and claims submission address should also be obtained. Verifying that the patient

Worker's Compensation

Insurance Verification

Today's Date: ____________________________

Patient Name: ____

Claim #: ____

DOI (Date of Injury): ______________________________

Insurance co.:____

Adjuster Name:____

Adjuster's phone number/ext.____

Adjuster's FAX:____

UR dept phone number:____

UR dept FAX:____

Has the claim been approved? (Verify the claim is active and open) Y/N

Claims Address:

____

____

____

Verified by: _____________________

Personal Injury
INSURANCE VERIFICATION

Today's Date: ______________

Patient Name: ______________________________

DOI (Date of Injury): ________________________

Patient's Insurance Information

Is there med-pay coverage? ____________________

If yes, how much (they may not tell you) $________

If yes, is it excess to their primary health insurance? _______

Adjuster's Name & Tel #: ___________________________
Fax # _______________________

Claim #: ______________________

Address to submit claims: __________________________

____

Verified By: ________________

If the patient does not have med-pay, you will need to see if the patient has regular health insurance coverage. Additionally, you will need to get a signed lien from the patient's attorney (have the patient sign one even if they do not YET have an attorney and keep it on file). Remember-3rd party liens are highly discouraged-they are a huge gamble.

has straight med-pay versus excess is also important. Remember that if the patient does have excess med-pay, one must also verify their health insurance since it will be the primary insurance billed prior to the med-pay (more on this in the PI section). If the patient has no health insurance, have them sign a quick statement to that affect. Although one should ask what the med-pay limit is on the patient's policy during the verification call, they often will not tell. Ask the patient if they know. They will receive a letter in the mail after opening their claim that reiterates the benefits and limitations of their med-pay policy, so they should know within a couple of weeks of opening the claim what the limit is, if they don't already. One should find out if any of the benefits have been used, to more accurately determine what's remaining. A sample PI verification form is on the previous page.

Your practice's insurance system should include, at this point, entering the patient's information into your practice management software (PMS) including their personal and insurance information for billing. If there is a notes section associated with a patient's account, it is *highly* recommended to use it for insurance tracking purposes, starting now. Summarizing the patient's insurance benefits should be first in the notes section. Subsequent verifications would go above the old. A typical summary would look like this:

4/30/08—TA (initials of verifier)
$250 DED/$34.28 met
12 visits/cal yr
Max $25/visit

This way, when working in the patient's account for follow-up, billing, payment posting, etc. the patient's benefits status is quickly available. In addition, in this same notes section, start keeping notes, in date order. Notes will include authorization information from adjusters and correspondence with insurance companies regarding claims or payments, etc. It is much more efficient to keep this information in the practice management system, with the patient record, than in a separate file. This places follow-up information in one place making it easier, more efficient, and follow-up more likely.

Case Studies

1. **Hearing that Ellen H.,** a newly-scheduled patient who was recently involved in an auto accident and has med-pay, we are happy to have a new solid case. To be certain of the details, we find out the total damages, what other care has been given so far and how much med-pay is still available. The staff learns that it was only a glorified fender bender, that the patient was taken to the hospital via ambulance, had MRIs and other costly diagnostic tests and has already seen a chiropractor for the past three months. We then find out that her med-pay is long-maxed, and since the case cannot handle any more medical bills even though she has an attorney, we decide not to treat the patient on a PI lien since the likelihood of getting paid is slim-to-none once the case goes to settle. Instead, the patient's health insurance is used for payment removing the worry about the unlikely future PI payment at all.

2. **Mary C.** was in an auto accident. After verifying she had med-pay and that none of it had been used yet, we treated her and were paid effortlessly for three months until her insurance began questioning the medical necessity of the care. After providing well-documented progress as a result of the care, we were able to continue treating her and be paid for all services for the next three months until she was released from treatment.

When the patient has no acupuncture benefits

The patient will have to pay cash at the time of service. Some of the insurance companies that you are contracted with have a "discount plan" for patients who have a company's insurance plan but without acupuncture benefits. Often, an in-network practitioner has contractually agreed to accept a discounted rate for services for plans without acupuncture benefits. Some companies who have this are Aetna (called the "Aetna Natural Alternatives" discount plan), Blue Shield, Blue Cross, Great West, Pacificare (aka, "My Life Path and Healthy Roads"). Through American Specialty Health (ASH) there is a "Health Net Well Rewards" discount policy; OptumHealth provides a discount program as well. You will need to figure out what these discounted rates are in advance, so that when you verify insurance and they tell you they have the "Healthy

Roads" discount plan (for example) you know what your office rates are. It should also be noted that just because a patient is covered by an insurance company with *no* acupuncture coverage, it doesn't *automatically* mean that they have one of these discount plans. During the verification process, if you are told there are no acupuncture benefits, you should inquire if there are any discount programs. To determine the discounted rates, review each of the discount programs' rules. Some have mandated fees a practitioner must charge whereas others require one to give, for example, 20% off of the regular fees. Remember that the "regular fees" are not necessarily your discounted cash rates. Regular fees (as if you were billing an insurance company) might be an acupuncture charge plus a therapy done in conjunction with the needling and so a 20% discount off of those may yield a rate just below the discounted cash rate. As a general rule, the discount should be slightly less than a practitioner's cash rates, in our opinions, so that the patient feels like they are getting a good deal and some benefit from their insurance.

Changing information with insurance companies

Avoid this like the plague!! If you must move or get/change a taxpayer ID number (TIN), you need to know the following:

- It is a royal pain and you must be diligent in making these changes. It can take years to get updated, as shocking as that sounds, so your diligence is necessary to mitigate this.
- With ASH, you can go online and change your address. It can take 30-60 days to complete, so be mindful of this. Since they are technically responsible for informing all insurance companies they contract with (Blue Cross, Cigna, Health Net, Aetna), it can create further delays in updating your information. We recommend you do the following:
  1. Always, always write a general notification of your address or TIN change info. State the effective date, the OLD information and the NEW information (make sure the new stands out more than the old). Then, in either case, you will need to attach your updated W-9. Make multiple copies of these two things, attach them and send them with all claims from now to

eternity (or until they actually make the change). We are serious about this; continue to do this for possibly months.
2. If you are online using any of the other insurance companies and can submit your changes through their website, you should. This, hopefully will substantially reduce the time it takes to get your changes to go through.
3. Remember to also update your national provider identifier (NPI) information. Log on to the NPPES website and follow the prompts to make the necessary changes.

Steps to take when a claim is denied due to misinformation received by the insurance company:

1. First, figure out the exact reason for the denial. Only once you know the specific reason, can you begin to figure out the solution. Scrutinize the explanation of benefits (EOB) for this, if the explanation makes no sense, call and ask.
2. If you discover that the reason for the denial is in direct conflict with information previously given to you by the insurance company, you can, if possible, resubmit the claim with updated or corrected information that would now make it acceptable to the insurance company.
3. If the reason is not something that can be corrected and resubmitted, e.g. there actually is *no* acupuncture coverage at all, you don't have much recourse. As annoying as it is to be told wrong information, they are very certain to always read the disclaimer that "benefits quoted are not a guarantee of payment..." which gets them off the hook for these matters. You can, as a last resort, call and plead your issue with the insurance company citing when you called, who you spoke to, and the reference number you were given when you were misinformed. All the more reason to get your claims in quickly, figure out the reason for any unpaid claims immediately before the patient is on the hook for too many visits which can cause them a hardship, and keep them from coming back to see you.
4. In some cases, a patient who feels very wronged by misinformation given out by their insurance company has the option of filing an appeal/grievance with their insurance company. This is a battle they can choose to fight but most likely, due to the disclaimer, isn't frequently won. Remember, the insured (patient) has much more power than you, the practitioner. The patient pays the premiums, they are their customer. They are much more likely to win any battle to be fought and should therefore be the ones to forge ahead with an issue as opposed to you.

Dealing with companies that are not forthright

This may come as a surprise, but sometimes insurance companies will not be forthright with information. Actually, you will be quoted 'misinformation' which is cleverly handled by insurance companies with their disclaimer they read prior to quoting benefits that says: "Benefits quoted are not a guarantee of payment, payment will be determined at the time the claim is received and according to the plan provisions at the time of service, etc."

So, how do you deal with denied insurance claims when you have received 'misinformation?' Try to be proactive at the onset. First of all, when verifying benefits, get the date of the call, note the customer service agent's name, and get a reference number for the call. Whenever a call is handled by an insurance company, their customer service software assigns a reference number. Getting this number greatly speeds any potential follow-up calls. Take note of this number when you verify insurance. Make sure the benefits being quoted *sound right*. The authors cannot tell how many times we have called to verify benefits and been connected with, let us say, someone not playing with a full deck and quoted outrageous benefits that did not sound right at all. You can ask to speak to a supervisor. If this is not effective, you may want to call back and speak to someone else. It is not uncommon to call back a couple of times until matching verifications are quoted. This may sound like a pain, and it is, but it is worth it in the end.

Even though everything has been done to verify the correct benefits, claims may still be denied for various reasons. Unfortunately, due to the disclaimer quoted when the benefits were verified, there are limitations in what can be done to dispute denials. Certainly *try* to fight this by cit-

Case Study

John G. is a new practitioner and was asked at a party if he accepted insurance. With little hesitation he replied that he did, even though he had never done it before. After that patient was seen a week later, John made a copy of their insurance card and, after figuring out some of the process of insurance billing, he submitted a proper CMS-1500. After four months, he realized he never did receive a check from the insurance company. Does he have any recourse? What could John have done to ensure payment?

ing whom you spoke with along with the reference number for the verification call and say they said acupuncture was covered and see if this makes a difference. Getting the patient involved can be very useful. Ask them to call their insurance stating that they misquoted their provider and so now they are financially responsible. Remember, the insurance company's loyalty is to the premium payer—the patient—not to the provider. The patient carries more weight and can sometimes get better results, in difficult situations, than a provider when an insurance company has grossly misquoted benefits or made other mistakes.

With regards to workers' compensation cases, there is some recourse if the insurance company messes with the provider. First, always get authorization before initiating a course of acupuncture treatment, *in writing*. In California, you must get authorization from the adjuster or review company prior to rendering treatment anyway, so *get it in writing*. If you do not, you run the risk of not getting paid. Often times, adjusters will verbally give you authorization over the phone, after which, any number of things can happen:

- They leave the company and the new adjuster doesn't see any record of that authorization so they won't pay the claim(s).
- An adjuster may forget they ever gave an authorization, didn't make any notes and, therefore, won't be paying the claim(s).
- A new adjuster may be assigned to the claim—one who goes by a different set of rules and doesn't think the patient should have acupuncture, etc. and so no claims will be paid.
- They may claim they did not realize the provider was an acupuncture clinic when they gave the authorization and, had they known, never would have authorized the treatment (of course, when we call we say we are checking the status of authorization for acupuncture…it's repeated multiple times)—this is especially annoying.

These are all experiences the authors have had. So protect yourself and always get the authorization in writing. If they don't have anything to send, write a quick blurb referencing the conversation and that they have authorized x amount of visits, etc. Fax it to them for a signature and request it be sent back. Hold firm to this procedure so you don't get burned. Another good reason for doing this is once the bills are being processed by bill review, they may not have a record of the authorization and deny the claims for lack of it. Only when the provider has it in writing, can the claim be resubmitted with a copy of the authorization as proof, which cannot be argued.

If the workers compensation company still refuses to pay the claim(s), a few of the following things can still be attempted:

1. Have the patient call and inquire about why their provider hasn't been paid.
2. Call the adjuster's supervisor explaining how you had authorization in advance of treatment and so there is no reason why your claims shouldn't be paid.
3. Call the patient's attorney, if they have one, and see if they can apply pressure for you.
4. File a Workers' Compensation Lien

A Workers' Compensation Lien (work comp lien) is a medical lien attached to a workers' compensation claim. If you are unable to get your bills paid, your last option is to file a work comp lien. You complete this lien on-line and file it with the local work comp appeals board and it gets attached to the patient's work comp claim. When the claim is finally settled (this may take years) the medical bill will be considered as part of the final settlement. Medical necessity (preauthorization) for the treatment must have been established for the bill to

Note

In California, the Work Comp Board has adopted new, automated means of filing liens. The good news is that you no longer need the patient to sign it in advance, the bad news is that the new automated EAMS system is extremely painful until you figure it out. To file a work comp lien, you need only complete the on-line form and submit it with all stipulated documentation. To find the lien, go to: http://www.dir.ca.gov/dwc/forms.html and search for the 'notice and request for allowance of lien' form. Other state's laws may differ, so it's a good idea to find out the rules for these liens in advance.

be considered. This is, however, the final safety net for getting paid on a worker's comp claim. Part of the work comp lien filing process includes sending a copy of the completed lien to the worker compensation carrier, which in some cases prompts them to pay your bills as well. Since filing a lien requires copies of authorizations and outstanding balances, this is a good time to reiterate to the payer that the provider has the right to treat and get paid. The lien indicates that you are serious about getting paid and are going to see this through to the bitter end. Since it becomes inevitable to pay, it is possible to receive payment just by filing and sending the lien to the workers compensation payer.

When the Patient Arrives 4

Checklist for Chapter 4: When the Patient Arrives

- If a new patient:
  - — Get signature on an informed consent form
  - — Get signature on a privacy practices form for HIPAA compliance
  - — If required by your malpractice insurance, have the patient sign an arbitration agreement
  - — Get a copy of their driver's license
  - — Get a copy of their insurance card on both sides
  - — Have the patient sign an assignment of benefits form
  - — Create a new patient folder
  - — Have patient fill out a new patient intake form
  - — Have patient fill out a proper outcomes assessment
  - — Give the patient a fee schedule
  - — If patient is a personal injury case, a specific personal injury questionnaire should be filled out, med-pay coverage verified, a copy of the accident report placed in the file, and an Attorney Lien signed
  - — If the patient is a workers' compensation patient, they should fill out a specific workers' comp questionnaire; verify their authorization if not already done
  - — As a provider, do an appropriate history and exam
  - — Chart history and exam properly, establish a TCM diagnosis, a differential and biomedical diagnosis, and a treatment plan
- If a returning patient:
  - — Make sure nothing has changed in the patient's information
  - — Determine that nothing has happened to their benefits such as using them with another acupuncturist, a new benefits term, or change of policy
  - — Do proper charting, including a brief history with changes from last treatment, exams, and new treatment plan
  - — Re-examine the patient at proper intervals including a follow-up outcomes assessment

Below are the things needed from a new patient upon arrival, depending on the type of case. Also, it is highly recommended each patient file is color coded to differentiate between cases: cash, insurance, workers compensation, personal injury, etc. When a patient's case type changes, a *new* file should be created. Each file should contain only information relative to its particular case type. Colored stickers are available for purchase at many office supply stores. One author uses labels from Jeter Systems since they offer all file labeling products, they last and do not easily fall off, and the company is very customer service oriented, organized, and prompt in order handling. The other author used a software program and labels from Smead that allow for printing on a printer any specific labels desired.

Insurance patients

- Take a copy of the patient's insurance card, both front and back, and their driver's license—these should be added to their file.
- If unable to get their insurance benefits verified prior to the appointment, it needs to be done as soon as the patient arrives.
- Office paperwork should include your office intake form, fee schedule, privacy practices (HIPAA), and assignment of benefits form.
- Once all paperwork is completed, make their file.
- Your fee schedule notification should state that insurance charges are *higher* than the cash rates (since you charge for all services performed when billing insurance). This informs them in advance, so that when they get their explanation of benefits (EOB) in the mail and see that you were paid more than your cash rates, they don't call you irate, wondering why you received so much more than your cash rate.

Workers' compensation patients

- The patient needs to complete a worker compensation specific questionnaire that addresses details of the work injury.

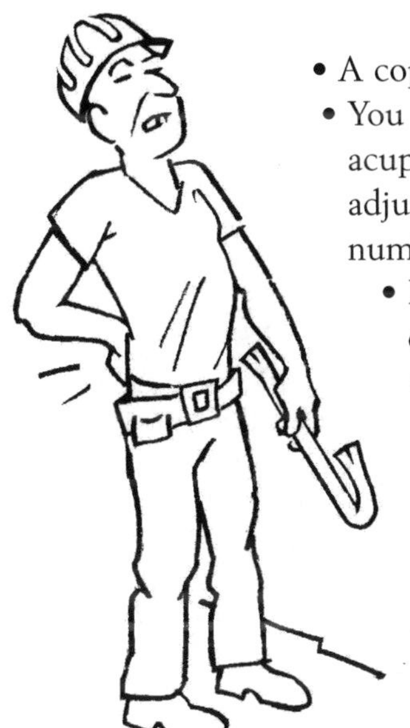

- A copy of the patient's driver's license needs to be in their file.
- You should now collect from the patient their prescription for acupuncture, their work comp payer information including the adjuster's name and contact information, the patient's claim number, and date of injury (DOI).
- If the patient has an attorney, this information should be obtained.
- A notification of fees and HIPAA form should also be signed and filed.
- The patient should complete the appropriate outcome assessments/pain questionnaires *on the first visit*. This establishes a baseline for comparing treatment outcomes to aid further authorizations. More on this in the outcomes assessment section under charting.

Personal injury patients

- The patient should complete a personal injury specific questionnaire that addresses the details of the auto accident or personal injury (i.e., slip and fall, etc.).
- Copies of the patient's driver's license, auto insurance card, health insurance card, and signed HIPAA privacy practices also need to be in the patient's file.
- They should also sign an attorney lien (even if they are currently unrepresented—more on this in the personal injury section).
- If the patient has an attorney, fax the signed lien to them for final signature and execution. If you choose to mail it, be sure to keep a copy.
- Call and verify if the patient has med-pay.
- Their health insurance also should be verified.
- If the patient has an accident report, a copy should be placed in their file. More discussion on why this information is important can be found in the personal injury section.

Paperwork

It is very important to have the proper paperwork in place to accept insurance.

1. **Patients must sign an assignment of benefits form** and it must be kept in their file. This authorizes the practitioner to bill the patient's insurance on their behalf and access their benefits for payment. See Appendix A for a sample of this form and more complete information regarding its use.
2. **Verify that patients have completed all necessary information** in your paperwork, including listing their social security number (SSN). Sometimes they do not want to give their SSN for privacy reasons. Unfortunately, this is often necessary for insurance purposes, even when they have a separate policy number, and so they need to give this to you if they want to use their insurance. Reiterate that you are a healthcare provider who is bound by HIPAA to protect their private information. This is not an unusual request and so hopefully they will cooperate. See the HIPAA section of this book for more information. For complete paperwork listing and form downloads prepared by the authors, go to www.acu-insurance.com.
3. **A HIPAA system consists of establishing specific privacy practices** for your office. There are two ways to conform:
   a. These privacy practices are given to all patients and the patient needs to sign a statement that they have received it.
   b. A copy of your privacy practices also can be located in your office in the waiting room or somewhere easily accessible and, additionally, by law, the patient can request a copy at any time. They must sign a statement attesting that they know where the privacy practices are located in your office.

   Whichever method is chosen, the signed statement needs to be in their file.

   HIPAA compliant forms are necessary for release of records and records restrictions. HIPAA meetings must be held with your staff and proof retained that they were conducted. Staff and practitioner education about HIPAA is paramount. Remember to educate new employees on HIPAA procedures and it is also a good idea to review your privacy practices annually in a meeting. Examples of HIPAA forms are in Appendix A or you can go to our website: www.acu-insurance.com.

Case Study

After creating proper systems for billing insurance, Janet's new receptionist submitted a CMS-1500 form for payment. Because of the systems, Janet realized she had not received payment after four weeks. She sent a tracer letter and resubmitted the bill. A week and a half later she received a response from the insurance company that the bill had been paid directly to the patient. What went wrong? Why was the payment given to the patient? What does Janet need to do now to get paid? Does she have any recourse with the insurance company?

4. **Health information intake forms.** Different health questionnaires for different case types should be created. For example, the cash and insurance questionnaire can be the same. Both ask for the usual information; name, address, date of birth (DOB), SSN, emergency information, health history, current health issues, and the like — don't forget to ask about blood borne diseases as they directly relate to acupuncture and tag their file to use caution with potentially contagious patients. However, for workers comp and personal injury type cases, more information is required and should therefore be added to these intake forms. Questions regarding accident details (date, time, place, description of incident, etc.) are needed to properly document the case as it relates to their symptoms. Who they saw after the accident, in order to request any medical records as well as coordinate care, is important to know as well as symptoms experienced before, immediately after, and since the accident. Knowledge of all of these factors helps show (and prove) a patient's response to treatment which justifies the bill and strengthens their case.

5. **Notification of fees.** Development of a general fee notification form that outlines fees for all case types; cash, workers compensation, personal injury (PI), general insurance, and American Specialty Health is important in order to notify patients in advance of the fees charged. See sample fee schedule on pages 25-26 above. The notification of fees should also address noncovered items or services by insurance, workers comp or PI (such as herbs, etc.). This is also the place to describe other services the clinic may provide such as massage therapy and what those rates are. The availability of any discounts offered (for seniors, military, students, etc.) should be listed as well. This would also be the place to describe any clinic and/or cancellation policies and associated fees. The authors also recommend letting patients know that your uninsured rates are discounted (only in California), or they receive a time-of-service discount (everywhere else). If at any time, their information changes, such as they have new health insurance or a new case (work comp or PI), they need to advise the office so the regular fees can be collected in addition to appropriately documenting their care relative to the new case type. Also, there needs to be a statement that recognizes the patient's ultimate responsibility for payment of their medical bills. Patients should sign this, acknowledging your fees and office policies.
6. **Personal injury (PI) forms.** Additional paperwork is needed for personal injury cases to protect your interests in the final settlement. The paperwork must include a PI lien (see boxed story below) and a personal injury policies letter/form (see sample in Appendix B on page 187). A lien is a legally binding document that the patient and their attorney signs, acknowledging that your bill will be considered during final settlement of the case. If you do not have an executed lien, the patient's attorney is under no obligation to pay you out of the final settlement. Although the patient is ultimately responsible for payment of your services, it is much easier to get paid from the attorney at the conclusion of the case than it is to track down the patient who has been given the money for your bill. More annoying is having the lawyer or patient try to negotiate a lower amount than they were paid for your bill. Save yourself: always get a lien signed! Then you negoti-

> ate directly with the attorney (remember to bill for all services performed). If the patient doesn't have an attorney, get a lien signed anyway. Sometimes the patient will get an attorney later, at which time you may need to send it to their attorney for final execution and if the patient is no longer being treated, it is difficult to track them down to sign it after the fact.

For a customizable lien, go to *www.acu-insurance.com*. If a patient refuses to sign a lien, then they will need to pay you cash since you are unprotected and have no guarantee of getting paid at the conclusion of their case. There is a lot more information to know on PI cases, so please make sure to read the personal injury section in the Introduction and

PI Lien Story

The following is a true story: Having not received any update on a case from a patient's attorney in over a year, despite numerous attempts, we called the patient to check the status of their case. We were told that the patient had been paid out a year prior and that they assumed we had been also. We waited to alarm the patient that they could ultimately be held liable for the bill and decided to go after the deeper pockets, the attorney. We told the attorney we'd inform the patient that they had never paid us and threatened to take their firm to court if they did not pay. Sending correspondence via certified, return receipt, we were guaranteed that he received our letters. Knowing that he was in the wrong to have dispersed all monies except for ours (which he had kept since times were tough), he called and worked out a settlement agreement, to which we held him. He did not want to go to court; it would make him look really bad. We would have had to name the patient in the lawsuit (since they too were signers of the lien) and he did not want the bad PR or have to face the patient. Since we had a lien, he was forced to play ball with us. Without a lien, he would have been under no legal obligation to work with us. Thank goodness we had a lien!

You should never take a case without a lien, this is the only protection you have to guarantee you are considered for payment upon settlement of the case. Without it, no one needs to pay you. You can take them to small claims court but it's time consuming, often not resulting in payment. You may get a judgment, then you can begin the fun of trying to collect on it. The system is definitely flawed in that judgments do not equal payment. Always protect yourself and your practice: get a lien!

NOTICE OF ATTORNEY LIEN (SAMPLE)

TO: Attorney
FROM:
RE: Medical Reports and Practitioner's Lien DOI:

I do hereby authorize the above Practitioner to furnish you, my Attorney, with a full report of his examination, diagnosis, treatment, prognosis, etc. of myself in regard to the accident in which I was recently involved.

I hereby authorize and direct you, my Attorney, to pay to said Practitioner such sums as may be due and owing him for medical service rendered me by reason of this accident and by reason of any other bills that are due his office and to withhold such sums from any settlement, judgment, or verdict as may be necessary to adequately protect said Practitioner.

And I hereby further give a lien on my case to said Practitioner against any and all proceeds of any settlement, judgment or verdict which may be paid to you, my Attorney, or myself as the result of the injuries for which I have been treated or injuries in connection herewith.

I agree never to rescind this document and that a rescission will not be honored by my Attorney. I hereby instruct that in the event another Attorney is substituted in this matter, the new Attorney honor this lien as inherent to the settlement and enforceable upon the case as if it were executed by him.

I fully understand that I am directly and fully responsible to said Practitioner for all medical benefits submitted by him for service rendered me and that this agreement is made solely for said Practitioner's additional protection. I further understand that such payment is not contingent on any settlement, judgment or verdict by which I may eventually recover said fee. If this account is assigned for collection and/or suit, collection costs and/or interest, and/or Attorney fees, and/or court costs will be added to the total amount due.

Please acknowledge this letter by signing below and returning to Practitioner's office. I have been advised that if my Attorney does not wish to cooperate in protecting the Practitioner's interest, the Practitioner will not

(continued on next page)

await payment but may declare the entire balance due and payable. Also, upon settlement of this case, I instruct you, my Attorney, to provide said Practitioner all medical records, billing from other providers, settlement amounts from insurance companies and third-party individuals and the proposed settlement split between all parties, upon their request. This information will be used solely for the purpose of the settlement negotiation for this case.

Dated: ______________________________

Patient's Signature: ______________________________

Witness: ______________________________

Print Patient's Name: ______________________________

ACKNOWLEDGEMENT OF ATTORNEY

The undersigned being Attorney of record for the above patient does hereby agree to observe all the terms of the above and agrees to withhold such sums from any settlement, judgment or verdict as may be necessary to adequately protect said Practitioner above named. Any settlement of this claim without honoring this assignment/lien will cause you to be responsible to this office for payment. The prevailing party in any litigation resulting from enforcement of this lien shall be entitled to actual Attorney's fees and court costs.

Dated: ______________________________

Attorney's Signature: ______________________________

Attorney: Please date, sign and return one copy to above Practitioner's office at once.

—Keep one copy for your records—

Appendix A. Establishment of personal injury policies for your office is very important. It is critical to have a form that outlines the policies regarding these types of cases that the patient signs. See Appendix B, page 187 for an example of a "Personal Injury Payment Acceptance Policy" that you might customize for your own use.

The front office staff should have new patient paperwork packets for the various case types made ahead of time. If you wait to pull each form individually at the time, you may forget a necessary form. It's also much easier when you are busy to simply pull a worker compensation packet out, for example, for a new patient. Make sure to set time aside each week for the appropriate staff to make new patient packets. There should also be a master copy folder (or file on your computer) that lists the paperwork needed for each case type and the forms for each case type. If this is not kept organized, forms will inevitably be omitted in error. This, of course, is never found out until you go to settle a PI case, for example, and realize you have no lien on file. Upon investigation, you find out all of your current PI packets don't include a lien when they should. Be proactive, keep the paperwork organized.

It is also recommended to make a new patient checklist that goes into each file. Review new patient files weekly and verify the checklist was done. Use this checklist to ensure all necessary information was obtained for the patient's case type. Additionally, include directions on entering pertinent patient data into the practice management software and any other things staff needs to review: copies of driver's license, insurance card and verification, a signed PI lien, if appropriate, and checking the health history for contagious diseases and having the file marked appropriately, etc. Basically, this is a reminder checklist for staff to ensure all information needed was obtained, things needing to be done were done, and so on. Since there are so many things that could easily be forgotten when it gets busy, this helps to avoid problems or catch mistakes before it's too late to fix them.

Using a calendar

An additional key component of a good system includes utilizing a calendar. There should be *one* common calendar that each staff member can access and notate on—presumably in an electronic format on a computer, ideally in your practice management software. The calendar can include notes to other staff members, reminders to do something, reminders to do monthly stats, etc. Notes in electronic format allow for responses to be written and the ability to be updated. A calendar is utilized thoroughly in this author's office. Notes to the staff, reminders to myself about follow-up, etc. are all kept on the calendar. One day each week is set aside for our staff meeting and so under the heading of "Meeting" anyone can notate a topic to discuss. Utilizing notes in the patient's account is also critical as well as being able to attach notes to an appointment, such as: "EOB received on Joe Patient and his insurance termed prior to his last DOS, please get new insurance info." Open communication, that is easy to document and track among staff in the office is crucial to ensure all tasks get completed. The best way to keep this communication is having outlets for them and a calendar system seems to be the best this author has found thus far.

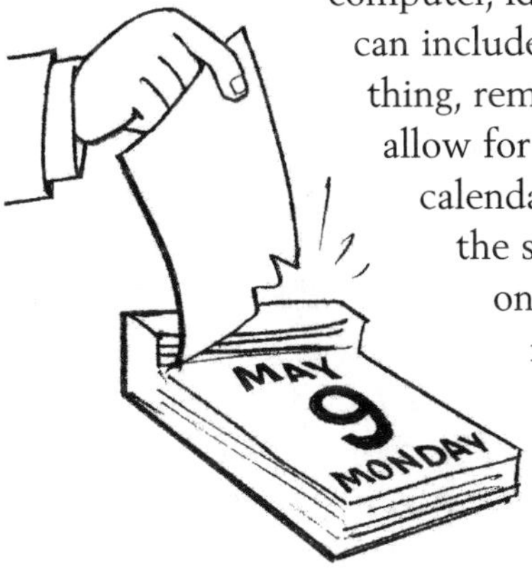

Summary

Whether or not you choose to accept insurance, systems are vital to the organized functioning of your practice. Below are some recommended forms to ensure your office has the necessary structure and remains organized:

1. Patient sign-in sheet (yes, they are still legal under HIPAA).
2. Daysheet summary—hopefully with whatever software used to enter patient data and visit information, a daysheet or equivalent which summarizes each day's transactions can be printed. A day sheet summary cover sheet should be created. This recaps the day and incorporates data from the daysheet print-out, the sign-in sheet (to ensure that the amount of people who signed in that day match the total amount of visit charge entries made into your practice software) and balances the monies collected in the format received, *i.e.*, cash, checks, credit cards, payer payments. The summary should also include any reminders to do at the

end of the day, such as: make change in your change box with smaller cash monies received, send welcome postcards or thank you cards for referring patients, send patient statements to any who left without paying that day, log data into stat log, etc.

3. Statistics log—to create statistics for the practice's growth. Three separate logs should be kept: one for each day in a month, one for each month within a year, and one for annual tracking between years. The log should include: patient visits, total charges, total collections, and total new patients at a minimum. One can add additional, important items to this log. Filling these fields in, after you have reviewed a daysheet also ensures that you haven't misplaced any of them…or the money that goes with them. There have been times when a day's stats were missing on the stat sheet which made this author have to look for the information. I had misplaced the daysheet and hadn't yet checked it or deposited those monies. It's just another way to check operations and prevent errors. Currently in business, using a dashboard for these statistics has become standard. A dashboard takes these stats and creates graphs from many of them and places them on one page so that many different areas of a business can be seen in one place. Using graphs makes it easier to pop out trends, but loses some of the specifics, but those can always be looked up. A sample dashboard is available on our website.
4. Patient intake forms—these should include: patient demographics, fee schedule acknowledgement by the patient, financial responsibility agreed to by the patient, HIPAA forms, arbitration agreement (if necessary by your malpractice insurance), and health history information. If the patient *does* have insurance, you should also make sure they sign an *assignment of benefits* form; this is a common form used to authorize the patient's insurance company to pay the provider directly. Copies of the patient's driver's license should be kept in the file in the event collections needs to be pursued and to guard against identity theft. Plus, it is nice to have a face to go with the file.
5. Insurance verification forms—this form should include patient's name, date of birth, insurance company name, phone number,

and patient's ID number as well as your Tax ID and NPI for easy reference.

It should address the following:

- Are there acupuncture benefits?
- If so, are they in- or out-of-network benefits? (If unsure about your network affiliation, ask them to check your Tax ID)
- Is there a deductible, if so, how much has been met?
- Does their plan go by calendar year or other?
- How many visits do they have per year, have any been used?
- Or is there a dollar limit per year, if so, has any been used?
- Is there a set copay or is it a coinsurance?
- Address to submit claims, and are there any special submission requirements with the claim(s)?
- Always document with whom you spoke, the date, and get a reference number for the call.
- The person who completed the form should initial and date it.

Verification forms should also be made for workers compensation and personal injury (PI)/med-pay cases since each requires slightly different information. The workers comp verification form should include the claim number, date of injury, insurance company name and address for claims, the adjuster's name, phone and fax along with the utilization review (UR) phone and fax. The same information should also be determined for the nurse case manager, if one is assigned to the claim. Ensuring the claim is open and active should be verified as well.

PI/med-pay verification forms include much of the same information as workers compensation. Since there is an adjuster assigned to these types of claims as well, the adjuster's information should be recorded along with the claim number and date of injury. The insurance company's name and claims submission address should also be obtained. Verifying the patient has straight med-pay versus excess is also important. Remember that if the patient does have excess med-pay, their health insurance must also be verified since it will be the primary insurance billed prior to the med-pay. If the patient has no health insurance, have them sign a quick statement to that affect. Although you should ask what the med-pay limit is on the patient's policy during the verification, they often will not tell you. Ask the patient if they know. They will receive a letter in the mail after opening their claim that reiterates the benefits and limitations of their med-pay policy, so they should know within a couple of weeks of opening the claim what the limit is, if they don't already.

6. Policies and procedures manual – A manual that contains instructions on how to do every task in your office, the correct way, is an excellent reference for employees. This manual should include original forms for copying, with what insurance companies the providers are contracted, any discount programs with which you participate and their rates, how to verify insurance, worker compensation, and personal injury cases, and finally, opening procedures in the morning, closing procedures at night, etc. Putting this manual together will help you to get and stay organized.

Special facts for California workers' compensation patients

If you are in California, **written** authorization must be obtained from the adjuster or review company prior to rendering treatment. If not obtained, there is a large risk of not getting paid. Often times, adjusters will verbally give an authorization over the phone, after which any number of things can happen. They may leave the company and the new adjuster doesn't see any record of that authorization so they won't pay your claim(s). An adjuster may forget that they ever gave authorization, didn't make any notes and, therefore, won't pay your claim(s). A new adjuster may be assigned to the claim (happens all the time) and the new adjuster goes by a different set of rules and doesn't think the patient should have acupuncture, so no claims will be paid. By the way, these are all experiences this author has actually had. An adjuster may claim that they did not realize you were an acupuncture clinic when they gave the authorization and, had they known, never would have authorized the treatment. This is especially annoying.

So, protect yourself and always get the authorization in writing. If they don't have anything to send, write up a quick blurb stating that per your conversation they have authorized x-amount of visits, etc., fax it to them and request it be sent back signed. Hold firm to this procedure so you don't get burned. Another good reason for this practice is that, once the bills are being processed by bill review, they may not have a record of the authorization and deny the claims for lack of it. Only when you have it in writing can you resubmit the claims with a copy of the authorization as proof, which cannot be argued.

A few more facts about workers' compensation: the adjuster *does* have the right to authorize treatment, independent of the review company and they can also override denials from the review company. Keep this in mind.

American College of Occupational and Environmental Medicine (ACOEM) Guidelines are used in California and a couple of other states as the basis for authorizing acupuncture treatment. They are very limited and do not address all conditions. To counter this, medical justification must be made to support your treatment and supported by research data. Citing reputable sources for conditions positively treated with acupuncture, along with utilizing outcomes assessment tools (discussed at length in Chapter 5) will help you to prove medical necessity and thus get authorization.

Having the correct procedures in place when a worker compensation patient comes to your office is vital to ensuring that you get paid. The first step in this process is ensuring that the patient has a prescription (Rx) for acupuncture from their primary treating physician (PTP) and that it has been authorized. In most cases, the doctor will have sent over a report referring the patient to acupuncture and the adjuster should have enough information to issue an initial authorization. Subsequent authorizations should be requested in writing by the acupuncturist. A progress report that clearly shows the patient's response to treatment should be faxed to the referring doctor, the adjuster, and the UR (utilization review) department or person. Sometimes the adjuster (or UR company) will review the request but may require a new Rx. The patient's involvement in getting a new Rx is usually necessary. If the request for authorization is denied, review the reason and submit an appeal if you think you can justify the course of care. Cite resources to support your treatment and the objective improvement the patient has made to date. Outcome assessment tools can be incredibly helpful in this endeavor. See the next chapter for details about and samples of Outcomes Assessment forms.

Clinical Aspects to Ensure Payment 5

Properly chart the patient encounter:

Subjective findings

- Include Outcomes Assessments

Objective findings

- Be thorough with your exam findings – insurance companies love this
- Include measurements

Assessment

- Include a differential diagnosis and a problem list
- Include proper International Classification of Disease (ICD-9) codes

Plan

- Include appropriate Current Procedural Terminology (CPT) codes
- Include a treatment plan

Education

Dealing with insurance companies is not necessarily about excess paperwork. It is, however, about proper documentation of a treatment. This documentation may involve a specific way of looking at a treatment. This does not mean that the companies are going to dictate where, how many, and how long you put needles in. It does mean that you have to explain what you did, why you did it, and that it is helping the patient. The technical term for this is "medical necessity." This means insurance only pays for medically necessary procedures.

To be medically necessary, the treatment needs to address a medical condition. Once that condition is dealt with, insurance will not pay for treatments any more. This comes into play with acupuncturists, because we would rather prevent a condition than treat it. Preventive care is *not* medically necessary and is not paid for by the insurance company. This means an acupuncturist can't bill for a year and a half for headaches without (1) showing substantial, continual improvement or (2) recurrence of the condition without treatment. In either of these two cases, charting and reporting needs to justify medical necessity since the insurance company may ask for reports to justify the treatments. Billing insurance without medical necessity is insurance fraud or at least very close to it.

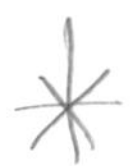

Of Note: Insurance companies have rules about what medical conditions they deem treatable with acupuncture. Even if you are treating a medically necessary condition, make sure *that condition* is covered by the patient's insurance.

Showing medical necessity may seem like a lot of extra work especially when it comes to charting. But here is a very, very important point: *Insurance does not require any more in treatment or charting than should be done anyway*. While using ICD-9 and CPT codes may be a little extra step, the rest of what insurance requires in your charts is exactly what should be done anyway. This means our charting should have thorough notes, not just because it helps our patients, reminds us what has been done in the past, and determines how they are progressing, but because it protects us. Despite some popular beliefs out there, acupuncturists do get sued for malpractice. And the only real defense in a malpractice suit is thorough chart notes.

Since proper charting is necessary from both a standard-of-care viewpoint and as a requirement for proper insurance paperwork, let's start by reviewing what constitutes good charting.

Proper charting

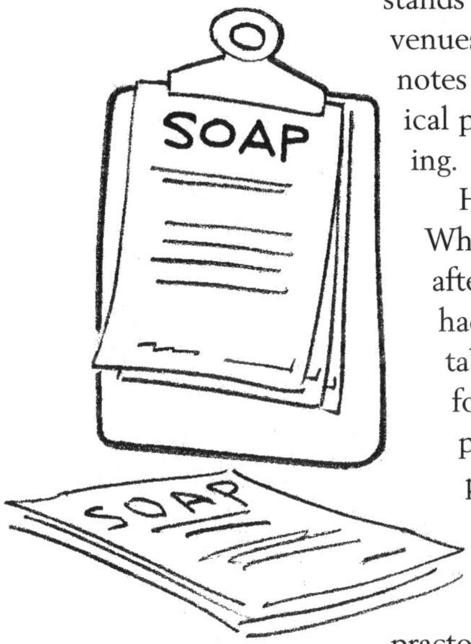

Charts are usually created using the SOAP or SOAPE system. SOAP stands for subjective, objective, assessment, and plan. Some venues are adopting SOAPE (pronounced "soapy") style notes which emphasize the education function of the medical profession. SOAP style notes are the standard for charting.

Here is a true story that happened to one of the authors. When working as a supervisor on a school clinic shift in the afternoon, a patient was passed from the morning shift. She had trouble with the treatment and could not move off the table due to spasms in her low back. After working on her for close to two hours using multiple modalities, the patient was no better. Luckily, another instructor on campus was a chiropractor and was asked to see this patient. He came in, saw the patient for about five minutes and had her up and walking soon thereafter. She was still in pain, but was able to get around. After that, the chiropractor was asked to write a chart note. He ended up spending about 20-30 minutes writing a note for a patient he saw for no more than five or ten minutes. When asked why he spent so much time on the note, he replied, "I have been sued for malpractice twice in my career.

General issues with charting:

- It is a major mistake to use the word "normal". This is a diagnosis and a very unclear one at that. What does "normal" mean? For example, "normal" blood pressure. could be defined as below 130/85, or it could be the old definition of below 140/90. Normal for a hypertensive patient may be 160/105. And when does blood pressure become too low? Generally, "normal" is a short cut that means nothing. When a person writes in a chart that something is normal, it indicates that it has been examined and the diagnosis is normal. What examinations have been performed? What if one practitioner thinks that normal means doing one set of exams and everything

...continued on the next page

continued from last page

is normal, while another thinks it means a different set of exams? What if one set has no abnormalities and the other does show pathology? The bottom line is: saying normal is a diagnosis that is probably not substantiated. Other points about using normal include:

- Instead of normal, use actual findings from exams, don't say heart sounds are normal; say heart sounds are dual with nil (or nothing) added.
- If actual findings are too complex when there are no abnormalities or to wrap several exams into one finding use the acronym NAD (No Abnormalities Detected). This is the opposite of a diagnosis because it basically says, "I didn't see anything wrong, but that isn't to say there couldn't be." Another acceptable acronyms is WNL (Within Normal Limits), but NAD probably offers the most protection against malpractice. **That said, actual findings are always better than a generic acronym.**
- Other words to avoid that are similar to normal include "OK" and "nothing."
- An exception to these rules are words that come straight from the patient. In this case, it is a quote and should have quotation marks around it.

- Don't mix up history, exam, and investigations or, by the same token, subjective, objective, and assessment. Common ways this can happen is within the history of presenting illness when describing the chief complaint, exam findings are mixed in. For example, the patient complains of pain on the leg 4 centimeters below the head and just anterior to the fibula. History would be the patient has pain on the side of the leg below the knee. Later would come the exam findings describing exactly where the pain is. Remember, history is from the patient, is subjective, and generally inexact. Exam findings are from the practitioner, objective, and should be very exact. Investigations are lab tests that are ordered by the practitioner and could include X-Rays, an MRI or CT scan, or blood work. The exception here is that investigations ordered by other practitioners are often included in the history of presenting illness (HPI).
- The biggest issue in regards to malpractice and insurance charting is not being thorough. The goal here is to answer all questions a reader of the chart may have. The best medical writers do this very succinctly in a small amount of space, but it is best to err on writing too much rather than too little.
- The first person should not be used in a chart. In a standard history and exam, the first person (using the words I, me, my, mine, myself, we, us, ourselves, etc...) is forbidden. Of course, the exception once again is a quote from the patient.
- Never, ever use white-out in a chart. If you make a mistake, draw a line through it and move on.

Both times, the other lawyer saw how thorough my charting was and dropped the case."

Subjective (SOAP)

Subjective notes include what the patient says or reports and do not include objective findings such as exams or investigations. Subjective findings, at least initially, are the equivalent of a full history which should include the following subheadings:

- age and sex
- chief complaint (CC)
- history of presenting illness (HPI)
- allergies
- current medications and supplements
- past medical history (PMH)
- family history (FH or FHx)
- drugs, alcohol, and smoking (in pack-years)
- obstetric/gynecological history (Ob/Gyn)
- sexual history
- personal and social history (PSH)
- occupational history (Occ Hx)
- review of systems (ROS), such as the TCM Ten Questions

Ongoing progress notes, obviously don't require a full history, only updates and changes in the condition are recorded as history of presenting illness. Let's look at each of these. The order of different subheadings is not necessarily standard and different practitioners move some of them around. Also, not all are necessary for every patient. Doing a sexual history can be quite embarrassing and inappropriate for someone coming in for a broken arm.

Age, sex, chief complaint (CC)

These three items are obvious bits of information necessary for treatment. Despite the importance of the chief complaint, sometimes called the presenting complaint (PC), there are many charts that don't get it quite right. Some pitfalls surrounding chief complaints are listed on the following page.

Issues with Chief Complaints

- Too wordy – A CC should be very succinct, just a few words.
- Too medical – A CC should be straight from the patient's mouth so we shouldn't use advanced medical language unless the patient has a medical background or a previous diagnosis.
- Too diagnostic – Unless previously diagnosed, a CC should be about a symptom the patient is experiencing, not what is causing it.
- Too specific – A CC is not the place to describe accurately where on the body a lesion is present; that is an exam point. In other words a good CC will say there is right low back pain. A not-so-great CC will say there is pain 3 cms to the right of L2-4.
- Too many – A CC should be just one complaint. Secondary and other complaints can be added in the problem list and expanded on either there or in other history sessions.

History of presenting illness (HPI)

This is also called the history of presenting complaint (HPC) and includes all relevant information about the chief complaint. There are, generally, two parts to the HPI: the narrative and the technical questions. The narrative should be a story about the complaint, for example the story of an accident causing injury or the story behind the last asthma attack: Like any good story it needs to include the who (usually the patient), what, when, where, why, and how.

The technical questions include the more technical medical questions about the chief complaint. These often use an acronym in order to cover all the relevant information. One acronym is OPQRST, which covers onset, palliative and provoking factors (what makes it better or worse), the quality of the complaint, referral of pain, severity, and timing and/or other treatments. Another one is OLDCAARTS which stands for onset of chief complaint, location, duration, characteristics (e.g. for pain whether it is sharp or dull), alleviating and aggravating factors (what makes the CC better or worse), related factors (such as activities of daily living) or referral (in the case of pain), timing or other treatments, and severity. Severity should be done using an appropriate scale, ideally something like the Visual Acuity Scale (VAS) but a simple scale of 1-10 is also useful.

Issues with History of Presenting Illness

- As stated previously, the most common error here is not being thorough enough.
- Not including a narrative of the CC. This means describing the experience of the CC from the patient's own words.
- Not completing OLDCAARTS or OPQRST.

Allergies

Stating allergies is of singular importance in charting and is probably not accorded adequate attention by many Chinese medical practitioners. From a biomedical perspective, drug allergies are incredibly important. From a Chinese herbalist's perspective, more general allergies are also very important. For example, it would be really useful to know if a patient were allergic to grass, as there are many grasses in our pharmacopeia.

Issues with Allergies

- Negatives are important and cannot be left out of a chart. Two acronyms that are frequently used are NKA (No Known Allergies) or NKDA (No Known Drug Allergies).

Medications and supplements

This is a list of what a patient is taking internally. The biggest point here is to include both pharmaceuticals and herbs and supplements. Research (Eisenberg, et. al., 2001) has shown that 72% of patients who go to both a medical doctor (MD) and a complementary and alternative medical (CAM) professional do not tell their MDs they are also using herbs and supplements. This means we, as practitioners, are the only healthcare provider who knows everything the patient is taking and can help predict ramifications.

Issues with Medications and Supplements

- A patient not taking anything should still have a negative under this heading.
- Doses of medications and supplements are often left out of Chinese medical charts. They are very important and can help determine any dangerous permutations.

Past medical history (PMH)

Past medical history includes any major conditions of the patient. In general, this means listing any surgeries, hospitalizations, major accidents, and major illnesses such as autoimmune or cardiovascular diseases, cancer, and diabetes. In addition, any past medical history that may be relevant to the chief complaint should be noted.

Issues with Past Medical History

- Not including negatives. If there is no significant PMH, a simple statement that there is no relevant past medical history should be charted.
- Not including illnesses that are relevant to the CC.

Family history (FH)

Family history usually includes heart disease, cancer, diabetes, major genetic illnesses, and anything relevant to the chief complaint. The relationship to the patient is very important to note. In addition, clearly noting if the family member has died and how old they were at the time of death is very important. Generally, FH just includes immediate family: grandparents, parents, siblings, and sons and daughters. Other members are generally not as relevant, though if connected to the CC, should be included. For example, if the CC is breast cancer, all female family members are relevant.

Issues with Family History

- The most common problem here is not making clear whether a relative is dead or alive and not including the age of death.
- Either too many or too few relatives are included.

Personal and social history (PSH)

A personal and social history should include marital status, social supports, living situation, religion/spirituality (studies have shown that active churchgoers live longer and are happier than non-churchgoers), and hobbies (with an eye to potentially harmful exposures). Some practitioners will place diet here, others place it under the ten questions under review of systems.

Drugs, alcohol, and smoking

Each of these substances, illicit drugs, alcohol, and smoking, have significant impact upon the health of a patient and need to be noted. Some practitioners will place this information under the personal and social history, however the authors find them to be so impactful on health, they deserve their own heading. When noting illicit drug use, the frequency and amount of use along with how it affects the patient's life should be charted. Illicit drug use can also include abuse of pharmaceutical drugs. Alcohol is one of the most common addictions. Charting it includes frequency, amount imbibed, and its impact on the patient. A common trait in all addictions is the desire to hide how much of the substance they are consuming and its consequences. Proper charting can take some insightful questioning.

A smoking history should include when the patient started smoking, how many cigarettes are smoked daily on average, and when they stopped smoking, if relevant. With this information, the exposure to cigarette smoke should be calculated as the number of pack-years. A pack-year is smoking one pack of cigarettes a day for a year. Twenty cigarettes are considered one pack. So if a patient smoked 10 cigarettes a day for 5 years, they would have an overall exposure of 2.5 pack-years. This information is very important in that it quantifies, relatively, the potential risks of smoking. Someone who has a 5 pack-year history of smoking is much less likely to develop health issues from it than someone who has a 30 pack-year history.

Issues with Drugs, Alcohol, and Smoking

- Not getting the relevant information either through improper questioning or patient obfuscation.
- Not computing the number of pack-years smoked.

Obstetric/gynecologic history (Ob/Gyn)

An obstetric/gynecologic history includes how many times the patient has been pregnant (grava or gravida), given birth (para), a description of menstruation, last examination and Pap smear with results, and if they have breast-fed (breast-feeding has been shown to lower the incidence of some cancers and raise others).

Sexual history (SH)

A sexual history includes orientation, the number of partners, use of barrier and other methods of contraception, and a history of sexually transmitted diseases. Obviously, this portion does not need to be completed if it is irrelevant to the chief complaint.

Occupational history (Occ Hx)

Occupational history includes a list of jobs that may have an impact on the health of the patient. Exposures become very important in this context and include such things as loud noises, chemicals, heat, smoke, physical hazards (such as a machinist being exposed to flying bits of metal or asbestos), vibration and repetitive stress, radiation, sun, and animals. Job injuries should also be listed here.

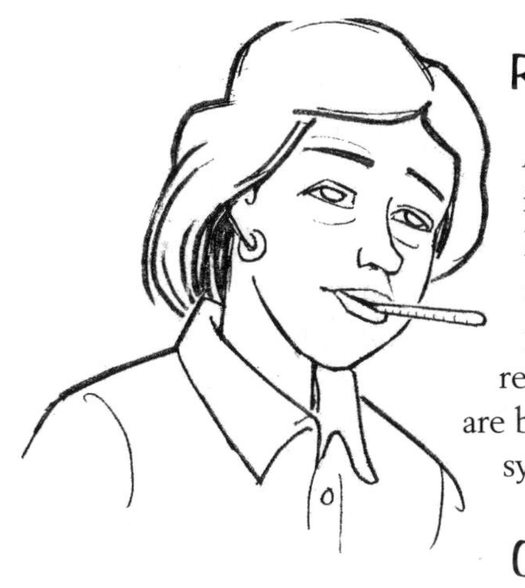

Review of systems (ROS)

A review of systems involves a couple relevant questions in each of the body's systems to get an overview of their health. In biomedicine, this may involve asking questions such as "Do you have a cough?" and "Do you have any phlegm, shortness of breath, or chest constraint?" for the respiratory system. In Oriental medicine, the Ten Questions are basically a good, if not biomedically complete, review of systems.

Outcomes assessments

Outcomes assessments are instruments to help determine the progress of a patient. They are usually specific questionnaires (though they can include some examination findings) relevant to the patient's chief complaint. They are given to the patient before treatment and again at various re-examination intervals. Good ones have been heavily researched for both validity (they give the information wanted) and reliability (they are consistent). Because of this research, they are considered to be very good indicators as to whether a patient is improving, staying the same, or getting worse and insurance companies like them for this reason. There are hundreds of different outcomes assessment forms and some insurance companies make them readily available to practitioners. Our website for this book, www.acu-insurance.com, will have numerous assessments available and there are also samples of several of these later in this chapter.

Using these forms is the best way to document progress with patients. Without them, it is much easier for insurance companies to deny claims. Using them makes it much more difficult for them to deny payment and allows us to successfully appeal such decisions. Filling out the forms may require some differences in how patient flow occurs in the office, but not much once the habit is created.

In order to use outcomes assessments successfully, a patient must fill one out when they first come into the office. The chief complaint needs to be determined and an appropriate assessment tool/form chosen. While there are some general assessments, such as the Measure

Your Medical Outcome Profile (MYMOP) or the Short-Form Health Survey, the more specific the instrument the better. Some widely used disability scales are:

- Medical Outcomes Study 36-Item Short-Form Health Survey (SF-36) – This is a general questionnaire that encompasses many aspects of health and is a good overview for almost any condition. The SF-12™ Health Survey is a component of the SF-36 that is easier to administer but not as thorough.
- Measure Your Medical Outcome Profile (MYMOP) – A very basic and simple-to-fill-out assessment where the patient decides which symptoms of their condition are important. The MYMOP has been favorably compared with the SF-36 (Paterson, 1996) and is much easier to use.
- Brief Pain Inventory – useful for any type of pain. This instrument includes a picture of the body so the patient can map the pain's location(s). There are two versions, the short and long form. The short is fine for most applications. There is substantial evidence as to the usefulness of this inventory (Cleeland & Ryan, 1994), (Tan, Jensen, Thornby, & Shanti, 2004). Other widely used general pain questionnaires include the McGill Pain Questionnaire, the Visual Analog Scale (VAS) or better yet the Quadruple Visual Analog Scale, the Clinical Pain Assessment, the Dallas Pain Questionnaire, and the Pain Disability Index (PDI).
- For assessing pain in small children the Wong–Baker FACES Pain Scale is frequently used and the National Institutes of Health (2007) uses the Checklist of Non-Verbal Indicators (CNVI) and the FLACC (Faces, Legs, Activity, Cry, Consolability) Scale. Others include the Riley Infant Pain Scale (RIPS) and the Modified Objective Pain Score (MOPS).
- Oswestry Low Back Pain Questionnaire – used for assessing the severity of low back pain and the progress of treatment. Several studies have shown this to be a reliable and valid method of gathering this information (Davidson & Keating, 2002). Other low back pain assessments include the Bournemouth Questionnaire, Aberdeen Low Back Pain Scale, Chronic Disability Index of

Waddell and Main for Patients with Low Back Pain, the Low-Back Outcome Scale, the Quebec Back Pain Disability Scale (QBPDQ), and the Low Back Pain Disability Questionnaire.

- Neck Disability Index – A very good instrument to assess neck pain. Other neck assessments include the Copenhagen Neck Functional Disability Scale, and the Neck Pain Score of Jordan et al.
- Arthritis Impact Measurement Scale (AIMS2) – is a 13-page questionnaire to assess arthritis. It may be a little large to use on a frequent basis although a short form is available (AIMS2-SF).
- Shoulder Pain and Disability Index (SPADI) – is used for assessing shoulder pain and disability.
- The Lower Extremity Functional Scale – can be used to assess problems in the lower limbs.
- Headache Disability Index and the Migraine Disability Assessment Score (MIDAS) are obviously used for headaches and migraines, respectively.
- Hamilton Rating Scale for Depression – This is probably the most widely used assessment for depression. Another scale is the Zung Self-rating Depression Scale.
- Many, many others are available at www.acu-insurance.com.

Each of these outcomes assessments should be evaluated for use in your clinic. Whichever you decide are best, should be readily available as a patient comes into the office. A general search for research comparing different assessments should also be done initially and periodically with the goal to use the most accepted scales at the moment. Make sure any relevant research is kept, in case it is needed to support the use of one assessment over another.

A list of the assessments used in the office should be available to the front person and they should automatically give the appropriate one to the patient as they are filling out their initial forms.

Here are several examples of outcomes assessments. Each assessment has a specific set of instructions on how they should be used and administered. Please consult our website for links to the complete assessments and instructions.

Name: ______________________ Today's date: ___________

*** MYMOP2 ***

Choose one or two symptoms (physical or mental) which bother you the most. Write them on the lines. Now consider how bad each symptom is, over the last week, and score it by circling your chosen number.

SYMPTOM 1: ______________________________

0	1	2	3	4	5	6
As good as it could be						As bad as it could be

SYMPTOM 2: ______________________________

0	1	2	3	4	5	6
As good as it could be						As bad as it could be

Now choose one activity (physical, social or mental) that is important to you, and that your problem makes difficult or prevents you doing. Score how bad it has been in the last week.

Activity: ______________________________

0	1	2	3	4	5	6
As good as it could be						As bad as it could be

Lastly how would you rate your general feeling of wellbeing during the last week?

0	1	2	3	4	5	6
As good as it could be						As bad as it could be

How long have you had Symptom 1, either all the time or on and off? Please circle:

0 - 4 weeks   4 - 12 weeks   3 months - 1 year   1 - 5 years   over 5 years

Are you taking any medication FOR THIS PROBLEM? Please circle: YES/NO

IF YES:

1. Please write in name of medication, and how much a day/week

____

2. Is cutting down this medication: Please circle:

Not important   a bit important   very important   not applicable

IF NO:

Is avoiding medication for this problem:

Not important   a bit important   very important   not applicable

MYMOP. Measure Yourself Medical Outcome Profile

Neck Disability Index
Simply add the score from your answers to the questions below and check the sum against the table.

Raw Score Level of Disability
0-4 No Disability
5-14 Mild Disability
15-24 Moderate Disability
25-34 Severe Disability
35-50 Completely Disability

QUESTION 1: Pain Intensity
A. I have no pain at the moment. (0 pts)
B. The pain is mild at the moment. (1 pt)
C. The pain comes & goes & is moderate. (2 pts)
D. The pain is moderate & does not vary much. (3 pts)
E. The pain is severe but comes & goes. (4 pts)
F. The pain is severe & does not vary much. (5 pts)

QUESTION 2: Personal Care (Washing, Dressing etc.)
A. I can look after myself without causing extra pain. (0 pts)
B. I can look after myself normally but it causes extra pain. (1 pts)
C. It is painful to look after myself and I am slow & careful. (2 pts)
D. I need some help but manage most of my personal care. (3 pts)
E. I need help every day in most aspects of self-care. (4 pts)
F. I do not get dressed; I wash with difficulty and stay in bed. (5 pts)

QUESTION 3: Lifting
A. I can lift heavy weights without extra pain. (0 pts)
B. I can lift heavy weights, but it causes extra pain. (1 pt)
C. Pain prevents me from lifing heavy weights off the floor, but I can if they are conveniently positioned, for example on a table. (2 pts)
D. Pain prevents me from lifting heavy weights, but I can manage light to medium weights if they are conveniently positioned. (3 pts)
E. I can only lift very light weights. (4 pts)
F. I cannot lift or carry anything at all. (5 pts)

QUESTION 4: Reading
A. I can read as much as I want to with no pain in my neck. (0 pts)
B. I can read as much as I want with slight pain in my neck. (1 pts)
C. I can read as much as I want with moderate pain in my neck. (2 pts)
D. I cannot read as much as I want because of moderate pain in my neck. (3 pts)
E. I cannot read as much as I want because of severe pain in my neck. (4 pts)
F. I cannot read at all because of neck pain. (5 pts)

QUESTION 5: Headache
A. I have no headaches at all. (0 pts)
B. I have slight headaches that come infrequently. (1 pt)
C. I have moderate headaches that come in-frequently. (2 pts)

continued on next page

D. I have moderate headaches that come frequently. (3 pts)
E. I have severe headaches that come frequently. (4 pts)
F. I have headaches almost all the time. (5 pts)

QUESTION 6: Concentration
A. I can concentrate fully when I want to with no difficulty. (0 pts)
B. I can concentrate fully when I want to with slight difficulty. (1 pts)
C. I have a fair degree of difficulty in concentrating when I want to. (2 pts)
D. I have a lot of difficulty in concentrating when I want to. (3 pts)
E. I have a great deal of difficulty in concentrating when I want to. (4 pts)
F. I cannot concentrate at all. (5 pts)

QUESTION 7: Work
A. I can do as much work as I want to. (0 pts)
B. I can only do my usual work but no more. (1 pt)
C. I can don most of my usual work but no more. (2 pts)
D. I cannot do my usual work. (3 pts)
E. I can hardly do any work at all. (4 pts)
F. I cannot do any work at all. (5 pts)

QUESTION 8: Driving
A. I can drive my car without neck pain. (0 pts)
B. I can drive my car as long as I want with slight pain in my neck. (1 pt)
C. I can drive my car as long as I want with moderate pain in my neck. (2 pts)
D. I cannot drive my car as long as I want because of moderate pain in my neck. (3 pts)
E. I can hardly drive my car at all because of severe pain in my neck. (4pts)
F. I cannot drive my car at all. (5 pts)

QUESTION 9: Sleeping
A. I have no trouble sleeping. (0 pts)
B. My sleep is slightly disturbed (less than 1 hour sleepless). (1 pt)
C. My sleep is mildly disturbed (1-2 hours sleepless). (2 pts)
D. My sleep is moderately disturbed (2-3 hours sleepless). (3 pts)
E. My sleep is greatly disturbed (3-5 hours sleepless). (4 pts)
F. My sleep is completely disturbed (5-7 hours sleepless). (5 pts)

QUESTION 10: Recreation
A. I am able to engage in all recreational activities with no pain in my neck at all. (0 pts)
B. I am able to engage in all recreational activities with some pain in my neck. (1 pt)
C. I am able to engage in most, but not all, recreational activities because of pain in my neck. (2 pts)
D. I am able to engage in only a few of my usual recreational activities because of pain in my neck. (3 pts)
E. I can hardly do any recreational activities because of pain in my neck. (4 pts)
F. I cannot do any recreational activities at all. (5 pts)

THE REVISED OSWESTRY PAIN QUESTIONNAIRE

NAME ______________________________ DATE ____________

How long have you had back pain ______ years _____ months _____ weeks

On the diagram below, please indicate where you are experiencing pain, right now. Please complete both sides of this form.

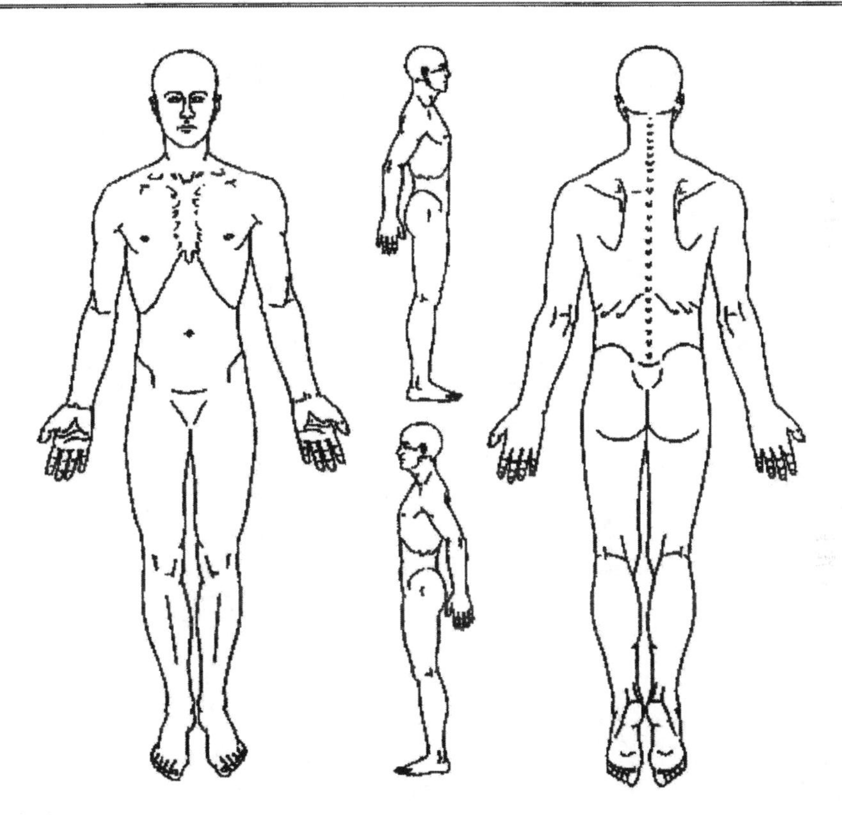

A = ACHE
P = PINS & NEEDLES
B = BURNING
S = STABBING
N = NUMBNESS
O = OTHER

The Oswestry Low Back Pain Questionnaire

Please Read: This questionnaire is designed to enable us to understand how much your low back has affected your ability to manage everyday activities. Please answer each Section by circling the **ONE CHOICE** that most applies to you. We realize that you may feel that more than one statement may relate to you, but Please **just circle the one choice which closely describes your problem *right now*.**

SECTION 1--Pain Intensity
A. The pain comes and goes and is very mild.
B. The pain is mild and does not vary much.
C. The pain comes and goes and is moderate.
D. The pain is moderate and does not vary much.
E. The pain is severe but comes and goes.
F. The pain is severe and does not vary much.

SECTION 2--Personal Care
A. I would not have to change my way of washing or dressing in order to avoid pain.
B. I do not normally change my way of washing or dressing even though it causes some pain.
C. Washing and dressing increase the pain, but I manage not to change my way of doing it.
D. Washing and dressing increase the pain and I it necessary to change my way of doing it.
E. Because of the pain, I am unable to do any washing and dressing without help.
F. Because of the pain, I am unable to do any washing or dressing without help.

SECTION 3--Lifting
A. I can lift heavy weights without extra pain.
B. I can lift heavy weights, but it causes extra pain.
C. Pain prevents me from lifting heavy weights off the floor.
D. Pain prevents me from lifting heavy weights off the floor, but I can manage if they are conveniently positioned, e.g. on the table.
E. Pain prevents me from lifting heavy weights , but I can manage light to medium weights if they are conveniently positioned.
F. I can only lift very light weights, at the most.

SECTION 4 --Walking
A. Pain does not prevent me from walking any distance.
B. Pain prevents me from walking more than one mile.
C. Pain prevents me from walking more than one mile.
D. Pain prevents me from walking more than 1/2 mile.
E. I can only walk while using a cane or on crutches.
F. I am in bed most of the time and have to crawl to the toilet.

SECTION 5--Sitting
A. I can sit in any chair as long as I like without pain.
B. I can only sit in my favorite chair as long as I like.
C. Pain prevents me from sitting more than one hour.
D. Pain prevents me from sitting more than 1/2 hour.
E. Pain prevents me from sitting more than ten minutes.
F. Pain prevents me from sitting at all.

SECTION 6 -- Standing
A. I can stand as long as I want without pain
B. I have some pain while standing, but it does not increase with time.
C. I cannot stand for longer than one hour without increasing pain.
D. I cannot stand for longer than ½ hour without increasing pain.
E. I can't stand for more than 10 minutes without increasing pain.
F. I avoid standing because it increases pain right away.

SECTION 7--Sleeping
A. I get no pain in bed.
B. I get pain in bed, but it does not prevent me from sleeping.
C. Because of pain , my normal night's sleep is reduced by less than one-quarter.
D. Because of pain, my normal night's sleep is reduced by less than one-half.
E. Because of pain, my normal night's sleep is reduced by less than three-quarters.
F. Pain prevents me from sleeping at all.

SECTION 8--Social Life
A. My social life is normal and gives me no pain.
B. My social life is normal, but increases the degree of my pain.
C. Pain has no significant effect on my social life apart from limiting my more energetic interests, e.g., dancing, etc.
D. Pain has restricted my social life and I do not go out very often.
E. Pain has restricted my social life to my home.
F. Pain prevents me from sleeping at all.

SECTION 9--Traveling
A. I get no pain while traveling.
B. I get some pain while traveling, but none of my usual forms of travel make it any worse.
C. I get extra pain while traveling, but it does not compel me to seek alternative forms of travel.
D. I get extra pain while traveling which compels me to seek alternative forms of travel.
E. Pain restricts all forms off travel.
F. Pain prevents all forms of travel except that done lying down.

SECTION 10--Changing Degree of Pain
A. My pain is rapidly getting better.
B. My pain fluctuates, but overall is definitely getting better.
C. My pain seems to be getting better, but improvement is slow at present.
D. My pain is neither getting better nor worse.
E. My pain is gradually worsening.
F. My pain is rapidly worsening.

DISABILITY INDEX SCORE: %______

Objective (SOAP)

The objective part of a SOAP or SOAPE chart note includes things observed, examined, or investigated by the practitioner. In other words, they are not reported by the patient, they are independently observed. Obviously, this includes pulse and tongue. But it also includes any appropriate western physical exams and investigations ordered such as X-rays, CT scans, MRIs, or blood work. Physical exam is not only necessary to treat properly – having taught physical exam class for many years, one of the authors makes a point that almost every exam can give useful information for treating with Chinese medicine – it is vitally important in order to avoid malpractice claims by looking for appropriate red flags. Physical exam is also very useful for determining and charting the progress of the patient's condition and treatment.

Insurance companies love to see thorough physical exams for several reasons. First, it indicates a diligent and conscientious practitioner. Second, it documents a patient's condition and how it changes with treatment. But most importantly, it documents the exam(s) for which the practitioner wishes to be reimbursed by the insurance company. So again, we should be doing an exam with every patient for medical reasons but it also helps support our insurance claims. Of course, all exams need to have objective measurements whenever possible and especially for insurance companies. There is a huge difference when supporting a claim between charting "range of motion improved" and "range of motion increased to 40 degrees from 32."

As far as charting goes, it is considered poor form to mix up exams and investigations. Each should have their separate subheadings and not be referenced in the inappropriate section.

For example, it is not good to say there were crackles in the lungs (exam), but the chest X-ray (an investigation) was clear, and the percussion note (an exam) was resonant. Here the chest X-ray is inserted in the middle of two exam findings.

Investigations ordered by other practitioners should be reported in history. Some insurance companies (both health and malpractice insurance) require that the pulse and tongue be examined and charted on each patient visit as a basic standard of care.

Assessment (SOAP)

Assessment involves the patient diagnosis both in biomedical and Oriental medical terms. And before the chorus of "but we can't make a biomedical diagnosis" rings out, here are the facts. In the state of California, it is the California Acupuncture Board's official legal opinion that since we can bill insurance and insurance companies must have a biomedical diagnosis, we must be able to biomedically diagnose (California Department of Consumer Affairs Legal Office). This same logic holds elsewhere: in order to bill insurance, one *must* have a biomedical diagnosis. If you are in a state where it is not in your scope of practice, then you need to get the diagnosis and the ICD code from the patient's medical doctor.

International classification of disease (ICD) codes

The ICD code is the heart of billing. ICD stands for the International Classification of Disease. The current version used in the United States is the ninth which is abbreviated ICD-9. There is a tenth version which is used in other countries, but should not be used here. And the 11th version is being readied and the profession is working to include TCM diagnoses!! An insurance company will *not* pay without an ICD-9 code. Period. Therefore, when submitting a claim to an insurance agency it must be included.

In the state of California, it is, at the time of this writing, legal for an acupuncturist to biomedically diagnose a patient. Therefore, they can use ICD codes without issue. The only guideline here is to diagnose only what you feel comfortable with. Diagnosing epicondylitis is probably fairly easy for an acupuncturist, diagnosing liver metastases probably is not, at least for most acupuncturists. A few other states allow biomedical diagnosing, but most do not. It is probably best, even in a state that allows biomedical diagnoses, to try and find out what the patient's medical doctor has diagnosed and use those codes.

If you are allowed or required to diagnose, it can be daunting looking at a huge code book. However, it is imperative that you decide on a code and use it. Having a code book is also a necessity. A practitioner who bills insurance cannot do so without either a code book or electronic version of one. Do not hesitate in spending the 80-or-so dollars on a good, easy-to-use code book. As technically savvy as the authors are, having a book on hand is much easier to use than electronic versions. In addition, a good medical dictionary is incredibly helpful in dealing with some of the names of these codes. Some hints on using ICD-9 codes as an acupuncturist include:

- Use pain codes. In general, insurance companies only recognize the benefit of acupuncture in treating pain and chemotherapy-induced nausea and possibly acupuncture used instead of anesthesia. This last one may be a bit of a sticking point. It is possible that some malpractice insurers will not cover acupuncture anesthesia, so check with them.
- Don't use ICD codes that are not related to pain. It adds a possible route of rejection. You can have all the information in your chart (and should), but don't use the code. The exception is if it comes straight from a doctor and then it is your discretion.
- Use the most specific code available. Codes should be used that describe the issue with the most accuracy. So if someone has knee pain, do not use the pain, unspecified code. Not only has it been retired, but there is a much more specific code available.
- Keep up to date with code changes. There are annual changes to the codes. Most won't affect us as acupuncturists, but every two or three years a new code book should be purchased and code changes should be checked annually. Keep an eye on our website for these changes at www.acu-insurance.com. Or join our RSS feed for immediate updates.
- Make sure that you are using the appropriate number of digits in the code. ICD-9 codes look like xxx.x or xxx.xx. For example,

724.3 is "Sciatica" and 717.81 is an "Old disruption of lateral collateral ligament." Some codes are only four digits and others are five. If you use a four digit code when it is supposed to be a five, the insurance company will reject it. A good code book will highlight which codes are five digits.

- Don't use accident codes unless there really was an accident. In the ICD-9, there are accident specific codes. They are all 800 series. These are used when an accident has occurred and describe things such as fractures, sprains, strains, and dislocations. When one uses these codes, the practitioner is risking that the insurance company won't pay. This is because if it is from a car accident, car insurance should pay for it (either through med-pay or a personal injury case), if it happened at work it is a workers comp case, and if it just happened relatively randomly, there is probably insurance somewhere (comprehensive general liability or "slips and falls" insurance) and it is a personal injury case. Insurance companies are paying for these codes more frequently, but they often get involved in the cases and ask for more documentation than usual. The test for using 800s is if the injury is acute. If a patient has ongoing, chronic pain from a previous injury, the 700 series or other codes should be used. If it is acute and due to a recent event, then the 800 series is appropriate.
- Know the codes you use. If you see the title of a code and think you know what it means, confirm it. Putting down a wrong code could be considered fraud. While this is a serious issue, the police aren't going to break down the door to your office and drag you to jail for an occasional screw-up, so do not hesitate to use the codes. What this does mean is: it is the practitioner's responsibility to know the meaning of the codes they are using. Using the wrong code risks rejection of the claim or a request for medical necessity. Both of which delay payment and causes issues with patients who receive the "rejection."

While ICD codes are vital to billing insurance, they are useful in other ways. These codes can be used for data mining. Data mining is the ability to look at large amounts of information to get trends and more specific and useful nuggets of information which can help run your office and possibly contribute to research. ICD codes are the beginning of this. For example, a good program can pull up each patient with a specific code and allow one to determine how useful treatment was. Combine this with the use of accepted outcomes assessments and you have a rather objective measurement of effectiveness. In other words, using ICD codes can be very useful later for many things that do not involve insurance.

Other parts to assessment

There are two other possible components to the assessment portion. These are a differential diagnosis (DDx) and a problem list. A differential diagnosis lists other possible reasons for the patient's condition. This can be as simple as adding a question mark in front of one or two alternative diagnoses or as formal as writing the main complaint and listing all the potential causes of that complaint. This is very helpful if the treatment doesn't go as planned. And it is very good training as to how to approach any patient's presenting illness. Insurance companies like it during their chart reviews as it shows a very thorough and conscientious practitioner. And that is pretty rare.

A problem list has all the issues or conditions the patient is dealing with even if the practitioner is not treating them. This is a very helpful list as a patient's condition evolves and should be available in a fairly static position in the patient's chart along with allergies and medications. These items also should be frequently updated as needed.

Plan (SOAP)

This is the part of the charting where the practitioner states the treatment plan. Now that the diagnosis is made, how is it going to be treated? This involves two parts. The first part is what the practitioner is doing currently. The second is what he/she plans to do in the future.

Charting the current treatment is vital. Being thorough and specific is extremely important as is recording how much time was spent on each treatment. Being thorough includes describing which positions the patient was in, which points were used in each of these positions, how long needles were left in, needle technique, and can even include which needles (brand, gauge, and size). If e-stim was used, which brand of machine, what frequency, which type of modulation (continuous, discontinuous, etc.), and amplitude (how high was the dial). All of this information is very useful for the next treatment or if someone else is going to treat the patient.

As far as insurance is concerned, time is a standard determinant of how much to pay as well as justification for the CPT codes used. It is absolutely crucial to put this in the chart. Time is one of the most important factors insurance companies look at for justifying billing and payments. All procedures, such as acupuncture and massage, should have the amount of time spent doing them written in the chart. In addition, any removal and reinsertion of needles should be charted as this impacts the ability to bill certain codes.

Current procedural terminology (CPT) codes

CPT codes are the current procedural terminology codes. They describe which treatments were administered. There are only a handful of codes relevant to an acupuncturist. Codes are broken down into three major categories which include evaluation and management, procedures, and supplies.

• Evaluation and management (E & M) CPT codes

Evaluation and management (E & M) codes are billable codes for assessing a patient's condition, both initially and during regular intervals of re-evaluation. Most insurance companies will pay for an initial E & M evaluation. There are five initial E & M codes. Which one is used depends on how thorough the evaluation was. Initial E & M codes can only be used once every three years by any one acupuncturist. In other words, if you see a patient once, bill an initial code and don't see them for another two and a half years, you cannot bill another initial E & M code. In the same way, if a patient returns after being gone for more than three years, one could charge an initial E & M code again. If a patient was seeing another acupuncturist in the same office within the past three years and now another practitioner is seeing them for the first time, an initial E & M should not be charged, but a re-eval E & M can and should be charged instead. The three year rule for charging initial E & M codes applies to the practitioner and anyone of the same specialty within the same office and does not apply to practitioners of the same specialty *not* in the same office. So if a patient were seeing an acupuncturist at a different office and just switched to you, it is acceptable to charge for the E & M code as you should be performing this service prior to any treatment.

Every acupuncture procedure, according to the CPT definition, includes a little time for a brief history and exam and therefore E & M codes should not and really cannot be billed for every visit.

Three criteria are used to determine which E & M code to use. While time is not one of these factors, it can be an indicator of the other three criteria. Initial E & M codes must meet all three of the given criteria in order to be considered at that code level. If the condition doesn't meet all three criteria it needs to be down-coded. These criteria are **history, examination,** and **medical decision making.** Three other criteria can help influence the code chosen but are not a main determinant. These are counseling, coordination of care, and nature of presenting problem.

History is broken down into four major categories. These are focused, expanded, detailed, or comprehensive. Most of our initial histories are probably in the comprehensive or detailed area unless we are focusing on a specific injury. Exams also follow this breakdown and our exams are generally detailed or focused. They are rarely comprehensive given the amount of training of most practitioners. Medical decision making is a little more complicated.

The five initial E & M codes are each described as "office or other outpatient visit for the evaluation and management of a new patient." See the summary chart on the next page.

In general, 99203 is the most commonly used initial E & M, and should form the bulk of your billed codes. Only rarely should 99204 be used and 99205 should almost never be used, even if you do spend the time with the patient, it is a major red flag to insurers. Both 99204 and

Initial Evaluation and Management Codes

All three major criteria must be met in order to justify a particular code. RVU stands for relative value unit and is used to determine how much should be paid for a given CPT code.

Code	History	Exam	Medical decision making	Typical face-to-face time (minutes)	RVU
99201	Problem-focused	Problem-focused	Straightforward	10	0.78
99202	Expanded problem-focused	Expanded problem-focused	Straightforward	20	1.49
99203	Detailed	Detailed	Low	30	2.28
99204	Comprehensive	Comprehensive	Moderate	45	3.86
99205	Comprehensive	Comprehensive	High	60	4.93

99205 are used when there is a risk of a prolonged or severe functional impairment, disability, or dying from the patient's condition (Collins, 2006).

When a patient is reassessed, a different set of E & M codes is used. These are often called re-eval E & M codes. These codes are used for re-evaluating patients on a regular basis. While a practitioner can use time as a factor for when to do and bill a re-eval E & M, a better criteria would be to establish an initial treatment plan that includes a re-eval every 4-12 visits. Re-evals have the same three criteria of the initial E & M codes, however, only two need to be met in order to bill a particular code. The description of these codes is "office or other outpatient visit for the evaluation and management of an established patient." See the table on the next page.

Again, most re-evals should be billed with a 99213. Only rarely should 99214 be used, and 99215 should almost never be used.

Another way to bill for a prolonged E & M is to use a separate code. 99354 is for an additional hour of E & M service. Officially, it states: "Prolonged physician service in the office or other outpatient setting requiring direct (face-to-face) patient contact beyond the usual service; first hour (CPT code)." This is an additional code to a regular new or established patient E & M code. If you still need more time, the 99355 is for additional 30-minute increments. 99354 and 99355 are not paid for by most insurances, but is paid for by some workers'

Established Patient Evaluation and Management Codes

Two of the three major criteria must be met in order to justify a particular code. RVU stands for relative value unit and is used to determine how much should be paid for a given CPT code..

Code	History	Exam	Medical decision making	Typical face-to-face time (minutes)	RVU
99211	Problem-focused	Minimal	Straightforward	5	0.27
99212	Problem-focused	Problem-focused	Straightforward	10	0.76
99213	Expanded problem-focused	Expanded problem-focused	Low	15	1.51
99214	Detailed	Detailed	Moderate	25	2.31
99215	Comprehensive	Comprehensive	High	40	3.25

Modifier -25

Unless an evaluation is performed without doing a procedure on the same day, the E & M code must have a modifier of -25 attached. In other words, if one evaluates a patient for the first time and treats them with acupuncture in the same visit then 99203-25 needs to be billed, not 99203. See more about modifiers later in this chapter.

Modifier -21

If you spend extra time with a patient doing a new or established patient E & M service, there are a couple of ways to bill this. The first is to add a modifier to the original E & M code. Adding a -21 modifier to an E & M code indicates a prolonged, continuous service. Many insurance companies will not pay extra for this modifier, and those that do will probably require additional documentation regarding the service provided. In general, it is probably better, if justified, to bill a higher code than to use this modifier (for example use 99203 rather than 99202).

comp systems, including California's. In order to justify their use, documentation must show how much time was spent on each service. The simplest way to do this is to note next to each section how many minutes it took.

• **Other evaluation and management codes.** Other E & M codes exist and acupuncturists can bill for them, however, they are rarely reimbursed by insurance companies with the possible exception of California's workers comp. These include telephone call codes (99371-99373) and team conferences (99361 & 99362).

Other E & M codes include consultation codes for new patients (99241-99245) and established patients (99251-99255). Again, these can be billed but are rarely reimbursed.

• Procedures

While evaluation and management are about history, exam, and planning treatment, procedures are about the actual treatment. Almost every type of treatment is assigned a procedure code. These may be broken down into modalities and procedures. A procedure is any therapy applied to a patient. These would include acupuncture, massage, moxa, etc. A modality is a physical object applied to a body in order to affect a therapeutic change. They can be unsupervised or need constant attention. In the case of an unsupervised modality, a practitioner may leave the treatment area for a short period of time, which is not the case in a constant attendance modality. Examples of a supervised modality include the use of a heat pack or infrared lamp. Constant attendance modalities, with the exception of manual electrical stimulation, are rarely used in acupuncture but include ultrasound therapy.

Units. A unit is the number of times a particular CPT code is used. Some CPT codes can only have one unit attached to them, others can have several. Any CPT code that has the word "initial" in its description is probably a one unit CPT code. An example of this is 97140 manual therapy (which may include massage) and is billed in 15-minute units. So if you spent 45 minutes on a massage, billing three units is possible.

Time. Another factor in billing is time. Units are usually, when talking about procedures, about time. Acupuncture is billed in increments of 15 minutes. While that may seem very straightforward, there is a quirk. A unit is achieved when half that time is reached. In other words, a full unit of acupuncture is reached when eight minutes of time is done, not the full 15-minutes. If we are billing for massage (which is billed in 15 minute units), 1 unit is reached at eight minutes and continues to 22 minutes of massage, a second unit is achieved at 23 minutes (15 minutes plus ½ of another 15 minutes). With these definitions, hopefully the reader can see how important it is to record the time spent on any procedure.

Acupuncture codes. The main procedures for an acupuncturist are the acupuncture codes. There are two sets of two codes each. The two sets are for acupuncture and acupuncture with electrical stimulation. Each of these is broken down into two codes, the first for the initial 15 minutes of basic history and insertion of needles and the second for an additional reinsertion for 15 minutes. Only one unit of the initial code can be billed on any given visit while any number of units may be billed for the reinsertion code. Just remember, billing for multiple units does not mean getting paid for multiple units.

Acupuncture CPT Codes

RVU stands for relative value unit and is used to determine how much should be paid for a given CPT code.

Code	Explanation	Minutes	Units	RVU
97810	Acupuncture without electrical stimulation, initial 15 minutes of contact with the patient.	15	Single	.90
97811	Acupuncture without electrical stimulation, each additional 15 minutes of contact with the patient, with ***reinsertion of needle(s)*** [emphasis added]. Must be used with 97810.	15	Multiple	.75
97813	Acupuncture with electrical stimulation, initial 15 minutes of contact with the patient.	15	Single	.97
97814	Acupuncture with electrical stimulation, each additional 15 minutes of contact with the patient, with ***reinsertion of needle(s)*** [emphasis added]. Must be used with 97810.	15	Multiple	.83

It is incorrect to bill 97810 with either a 97813 or 97814 and vice versa. In other words, a practitioner cannot combine non-E-stim acupuncture with E-stim acupuncture. If you start with a 97810 and do a reinsertion, even if it involves E-stim, you must bill 97811. And if you bill 97813, you must bill 97814 upon reinsertion, regardless if there is E-stim or not. The take-home message is: if you are going to do some acupuncture with E-stim and some without, start with the E-stim as it has a higher reimbursement.

An important concept here is that both 97810 and 97813 contain some basic history and exam within the code and pays more for it. This means you cannot bill an E & M code in addition to an acupuncture code on every visit; only on the initial visit and periodic reevaluations. Both 97811 and 97814 require a reinsertion. That means if an acupuncturist puts needles in a patient and then leaves the room for 40 minutes, he or she can only bill for a 97810 **not** for a 97810 and two units of 97811. It also means if a practitioner does 25 minutes of acupuncture without reinsertion and then cups for 15 minutes, he or she cannot bill for a 97810 and a 97811 because there was no reinsertion of needles and cupping is not considered acupuncture. In this case, they may be able to bill for a 97140, manual therapy, for the cupping, in addition to the 97810, and hope the insurance company pays.

Other CPT codes. There are many other codes that can be used in an acupuncture practice, though not all insurance companies will pay for each of these codes. Some insurance companies allow you to ask for what codes they will compensate and others need to be determined by talking with other experienced acupuncturists or through trial and error. This is why you should always bill all that you do, see what gets paid, and keep track.

Billing for massage is a somewhat controversial endeavor. A straight massage code exists (97124). The reimbursement for this is usually pretty low. Some acupuncturists prefer to bill another code for manual therapy technique (97140) because it pays more and yet the description still fits and is more widely accepted by insurance companies. Another code, 97250 for myofascial release, is not part of the CPT codes anymore but is billable under the California workers compensation system and should be used in that scenario as 97140 is not used in that system.

Other CPT Codes

RVU stands for relative value unit and is used to determine how much should be paid for a given CPT code.

Code	Explanation	Notes	Minutes	Units	RVU
97010	Hot or cold packs applied to one or more areas	Typically not paid by health insurance. It is payable for PI cases.		Single	.17
97012	Mechanical traction to one or more areas	Use when using a device to apply traction		Single	.46
97014	E-stim unattended, to one or more areas			Single	.45
97016	Vasopneumatic devices to one or more areas	Might be used for cupping &/or vibratory massage		Single	.54
97018	Parafin Bath		15	Multiple	.30
97026	Infrared therapy	Use for employing a heat lamp			.17
97110	Therapeutic exercise to develop strength, endurance, range of motion, and/or flexibility*		15	Multiple	.91
97112	Neuromuscular re-education of movement, posture, balance, proprioception for sitting and/or standing activities, and/or kinesthetic sense*		15	Multiple	.95
97124	Therapeutic procedure; massage		15	Multiple	.74
97140†	Manual therapy techniques, for example mobilization/manipulation, manual lymphatic drainage, and manual traction, each 15 minutes	Many acupuncturists use this code instead of 97124 when doing massage as it pays more and can be justified	15	Multiple	.85
97250	Myofascial release	**Only used in the California workers comp system instead of 97140**	15	Multiple	

* These are controversial in that they are generally considered physical therapy codes. In some states, including California, they may fall into an acupuncturist's scope of practice. Since they are controversial, careful documentation is even more important than usual.

† When using 97140 three things should be noted: what technique is used, location, and time. Of note: In the experience of these Authors, it has been helpful from time to time to add a modifier-59 when billing a 97140 code, for it to be paid.

Medical records. When a patient, insurance company, or other entity requests medical records, it is allowable and expected to charge for these requests. There are two codes that cover these requests. The first is an overall administrative fee and the second is a per page fee. Generally, one would charge for both, though certain state entities have their own dictated charges. For example, California evidence code (for lawsuits) dictates $24 per hour for administrative costs and 10 cents per page (Collins, 2009).

Medical Records CPT Codes

Code	Explanation	Units
S9981	Medical records copying fee, administrative	Single
S9982	Medical records copying fee, per page	Multiple

*Subpoenaed records are copied in your office by a copy service. You should collect $15 from them either at the time the subpoena is delivered or at the time of copy, no exceptions.

Tests & measurements. Depending on the scope of practice for acupuncturists in individual states, there are a slew of tests that could be performed in an acupuncturist's clinic. Each of the following in the next table is probably within the scope of practice in California and possibly elsewhere. While they may seem to be very biomedical, they can be very useful for Chinese medical patients. For example, knowing if a patient is pregnant or not has a large impact on acupuncture point choice.

Tests & Measurements CPT Codes

Code	Explanation	Minutes	Units	RVU
81002	Urinalysis nonauto w/o scope		Single	$ 3.60
81025	Urine pregnancy test		Single	$ 8.90
82962	Glucose blood test		Single	$ 3.29
87880	Strep A assay w/optic		Single	$16.88
97750	Physical performance test for measurement (eg. musculoskeletal, functional capacity) with a written report, each 15 mins	15	Multiple	$ .95

* 8xxxx laboratory codes do not have RVUs, just straight Medicare reimbursements. To distinguish these straight dollar amounts, the book includes dollar signs before non-RVU reimbursements.

California workers' compensation codes

California workers compensation is almost a separate system in their coding. Instead of 97810 through 97814 they use just 97780 for no electrical stimulation and 97781 for acupuncture with electrical stimulation. These are based on the old CPT codes. When the rest of the country changed to 97810-97814 in 2005, the California workers comp system did not. This means there are no codes for an additional 15 minutes of re-insertion and you can use more than one unit of time for these codes. At the time of writing this, there are proposals to update the California workers compensation system to the coding system used by everyone else in the United States.

Modifiers. Modifiers are designed to modify a CPT code where the procedure is essentially the same but circumstances are slightly different than the official definition of the procedure. Examples include taking a shorter or longer time with a given procedure or performing an evaluation at the same time as a procedure. Modifiers should be used when circumstances alter a procedure to the point where it may affect reimbursement. Or they can be for information only. Modifiers are two digit codes added to the end of a CPT code. The table on page 104 shows a list of common CPT modifiers used by acupuncturists.

Herbs and other supplements. There are HCPCS codes for items other than prescription medicines. While we can bill these codes, almost no insurance company will reimburse for them. The only possible exception may be health savings accounts (HSAs), some of which do pay for herbs and supplements. The A9150 code is technically for a nonprescription drug and this may be a gray area for billing. However it is often interpreted as "nonprescription item."

A9150	Misc/experimental nonprescription drug

Supplies. As above, acupuncturists can bill for needles using the Healthcare Common Procedure Coding System (HCPCS). Remember, however, billing an item does not mean getting paid for an item.

CPT Modifier Codes

Code	
-21	**Prolonged Evaluation and Management (E & M) Service**
	When face-to-face contact is greater than that usually required for the highest E & M level within a given category. Comment: Should be used rarely as reimbursement is iffy and almost always requires additional documentation. CPT codes 99354 & 99355 should be used for additional E & M services, if services were provided intermittently. Use this modifier for continuous patient contact.
-25	**Significant, Separately Identifiable E & M Service by the Same Physician on the Same Day of a Procedure or Other Service**
	Comment: This modifier should be used when an E & M code is used on the same day as a procedure or another service. Remember that the initial acupuncture codes (97810 & 97813) include a small amount of evaluation and management, therefore E & M CPT codes should only be used on the initial visit and intermittently, as medically necessary, thereafter. If a separate E & M code is used in addition to a procedure such as acupuncture, it must be modified with this modifier.
-50	**Bilateral Procedure**
	If a procedure's description doesn't state it is applied to both sides, this modifier indicates a procedure has been performed bilaterally. Comment: The American Medical Association (AMA) has stated the proper use of this modifier is to apply it on one line with one unit applied to the procedure and reimbursement should then include a bilateral procedure. However, some insurance companies prefer adding the -50 modifier to a second CPT *code.*
-59	**Distinct Procedural Service**
	This modifier states that a procedure is distinct or independent from other services performed on the same day. This can include a separate session or patient encounter, a different procedure, a different site, different injury. Comment: This modifier is used when an acupuncturist bills different therapies used on the same visit. For example, some insurance companies will deny a claim where an acupuncture treatment (97810) is performed at the same time as a manual therapy (97140). If a -59 modifier is used on 97140, it generally goes through with fewer issues.

A4215	Needle, Sterile, Any Size, Each
Comment: When using this code, it is recommended to only charge once. Reimbursement for this code is iffy.	

• Advanced billing concepts (ABC) codes

Advanced billing concepts (ABC) codes were developed by a company called Alternative Link, Inc. They were developed because the Common Procedural Terminology (CPT) codes were developed by the American Medical Association and are geared to MDs and DOs and minimally towards other healthcare practitioners including complementary and alternative medical providers, physical and occupational therapists, and nurses. ABC codes were created to help bridge this gap. While they are currently US government approved for use, no insurance company or entity accepts them for billing purposes. For this reason, they are not at all useful for acupuncturists today, and it is the authors' opinions to avoid their use unless they become more accepted.

• Time

Time is so important when billing insurance and so infrequently documented in acupuncture charts, it deserves its own subheading. Since many medical procedures are billed according to time, it is absolutely

The healthcare common procedure coding system (HCPCS)

The Healthcare Common Procedure Coding System (HCPCS) is another billing system that encompasses the current procedure terminology (CPT) codes. CPT codes are administered by the American Medical Association and are considered level I of the HCPCS codes. Level II of the HCPCS codes are a set of codes that begin with a letter from A to V followed by 4 numbers. They are administered by the Centers for Medicare & Medicaid Services (CMS) and includes quite a bit of overlap with the CPT codes. The level II codes also include codes for supplies that acupuncturists can bill for, but may not be reimbursed for on a regular basis. These include needles.

vital that time is charted. Examples abound. Acupuncture is billed in 15-minute increments as is massage. If there is no time noted in the chart, there is no justification for billing *any* of these CPT codes and the insurance company can and will deny your claim. In addition, insurance companies can request to audit your records more globally and *retroactively* bill you for a refund of previously paid reimbursements. This could amount to hundreds of thousands of dollars.

As an aside, just because an insurance company bills you for a refund, legally a practitioner may not need to pay it. If a practitioner is contracted (in-network) with the insurance company, they will be contractually required to repay the insurance company. However, if a practitioner is not contracted with a particular company (out-of-network), the law says the company cannot require a refund of previously paid fees.

Treatment plans (SOAP)

Up to this point under plans, we have covered what has been done for the current treatment. The next and final part of the plan portion of SOAP or SOAPE notes is a treatment plan. Treatment plans do not need to be elaborate. They can be as simple as "two treatments a week for four weeks and reassess" or "6-8 treatments and re-evaluate."

Case Study

After seeing a patient for six visits and receiving payments for five of those visits, Joanna, an acupuncturist, received a letter from the insurance company asking for justification of the sixth and all previous visits. The patient in question had an ankle injury but also asked for some help dealing with her insomnia. The chart notes clearly noted both conditions, but the only exam findings were pulse and tongue. After sending the insurance company a summary letter about the ankle injury and a copy of the chart notes for each visit, the insurance company responded by rejecting payment on the sixth visit and requesting their money back on the previous visits because insomnia was not a covered condition. Why did the insurance company respond this way? What could Joanna have done to demonstrate the treatment and progress of the ankle injury?

Insurance companies like to see these in chart notes because they show thoughtful herding of the patient through the treatment process. They are just good charting procedures.

In addition to acupuncture treatments, anything that requires further assessment or referral should be mentioned. This includes any future tests or investigations and follow up on referrals to other practitioners. Examples include, "Check blood sugar levels on each visit and HbA1C every six months" or, "Confirm patient has seen endocrinologist and received a report from the endocrinologist."

Education (SOAPE)

Education is the last heading when using SOAPE notes. It emphasizes the educational duty that every medical practitioner has towards their patients. One side of this is lifestyle advice and can include sleeping habits, diet, exercise, stretching, and relaxation techniques. The other aspect is to cover yourself for malpractice reasons. Every practitioner should have information sheets for various procedures they perform. Examples include instructions for the patient after receiving massage, cupping, gua sha, or moxibustion. It is just good practice to have these ready to hand to patients and to note in the chart when a patient has received them.

After the Patient Leaves

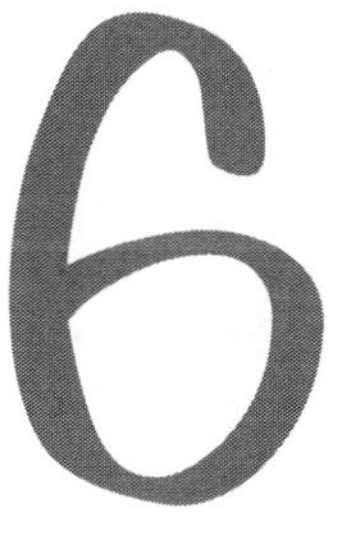

Checklist for Chapter 6:

- Prepare and submit a claim

  Use the CMS 1500 Form, or...
- Submit directly on-line
- Follow-up on unpaid claims

Preparing and submitting a claim

Hopefully your practice management software (PMS) has the capability of automatically generating claim forms for you. Whether you must complete them manually or review what your PMS automatically did, knowing the fields on a claim form are *mandatory* so your claim goes through without rejection.

Here we review, by box number, the mandatory fields on the CMS 1500 necessary for claim processing. CMS stands for the Centers for Medicare & Medicaid Services. The CMS 1500 is the form necessary to submit claims to Medicare and has been adopted by all insurance companies. It used to be called the HCFA 1500. All the numbers below refer to the appropriate box on the CMS 1500 form.

Figure 6-1: Sample CMS 1500 Standard Insurance Billing Form

1500

HEALTH INSURANCE CLAIM FORM

APPROVED BY NATIONAL UNIFORM CLAIM COMMITTEE 08/05

PICA | PICA

CARRIER

1. MEDICARE (Medicare #) | MEDICAID (Medicaid #) | TRICARE CHAMPUS (Sponsor's SSN) | CHAMPVA (Member ID#) | GROUP HEALTH PLAN (SSN or ID) | FECA BLK LUNG (SSN) | OTHER (ID)

1a. INSURED'S I.D. NUMBER (For Program in Item 1)

2. PATIENT'S NAME (Last Name, First Name, Middle Initial)

3. PATIENT'S BIRTH DATE MM DD YY SEX M F

4. INSURED'S NAME (Last Name, First Name, Middle Initial)

5. PATIENT'S ADDRESS (No., Street)

6. PATIENT RELATIONSHIP TO INSURED Self Spouse Child Other

7. INSURED'S ADDRESS (No., Street)

CITY STATE

8. PATIENT STATUS Single Married Other

CITY STATE

ZIP CODE TELEPHONE (Include Area Code) ( )

Employed Full-Time Student Part-Time Student

ZIP CODE TELEPHONE (Include Area Code) ( )

9. OTHER INSURED'S NAME (Last Name, First Name, Middle Initial)

10. IS PATIENT'S CONDITION RELATED TO:

11. INSURED'S POLICY GROUP OR FECA NUMBER

a. OTHER INSURED'S POLICY OR GROUP NUMBER

a. EMPLOYMENT? (Current or Previous) YES NO

a. INSURED'S DATE OF BIRTH MM DD YY SEX M F

b. OTHER INSURED'S DATE OF BIRTH MM DD YY SEX M F

b. AUTO ACCIDENT? YES NO PLACE (State)

b. EMPLOYER'S NAME OR SCHOOL NAME

c. EMPLOYER'S NAME OR SCHOOL NAME

c. OTHER ACCIDENT? YES NO

c. INSURANCE PLAN NAME OR PROGRAM NAME

d. INSURANCE PLAN NAME OR PROGRAM NAME

10d. RESERVED FOR LOCAL USE

d. IS THERE ANOTHER HEALTH BENEFIT PLAN? YES NO *If yes*, return to and complete item 9 a-d.

READ BACK OF FORM BEFORE COMPLETING & SIGNING THIS FORM.

12. PATIENT'S OR AUTHORIZED PERSON'S SIGNATURE I authorize the release of any medical or other information necessary to process this claim. I also request payment of government benefits either to myself or to the party who accepts assignment below.

SIGNED ____ DATE ____

13. INSURED'S OR AUTHORIZED PERSON'S SIGNATURE I authorize payment of medical benefits to the undersigned physician or supplier for services described below.

SIGNED ____

PATIENT AND INSURED INFORMATION

14. DATE OF CURRENT: MM DD YY ILLNESS (First symptom) OR INJURY (Accident) OR PREGNANCY(LMP)

15. IF PATIENT HAS HAD SAME OR SIMILAR ILLNESS. GIVE FIRST DATE MM DD YY

16. DATES PATIENT UNABLE TO WORK IN CURRENT OCCUPATION FROM MM DD YY TO MM DD YY

17. NAME OF REFERRING PROVIDER OR OTHER SOURCE 17a. 17b. NPI

18. HOSPITALIZATION DATES RELATED TO CURRENT SERVICES FROM MM DD YY TO MM DD YY

19. RESERVED FOR LOCAL USE

20. OUTSIDE LAB? YES NO $ CHARGES

21. DIAGNOSIS OR NATURE OF ILLNESS OR INJURY (Relate Items 1, 2, 3 or 4 to Item 24E by Line)

1. ___ . ___ 3. ___ . ___

2. ___ . ___ 4. ___ . ___

22. MEDICAID RESUBMISSION CODE ORIGINAL REF. NO.

23. PRIOR AUTHORIZATION NUMBER

	24. A. DATE(S) OF SERVICE From MM DD YY To MM DD YY	B. PLACE OF SERVICE	C. EMG	D. PROCEDURES, SERVICES, OR SUPPLIES (Explain Unusual Circumstances) CPT/HCPCS MODIFIER	E. DIAGNOSIS POINTER	F. $ CHARGES	G. DAYS OR UNITS	H. EPSDT Family Plan	I. ID. QUAL.	J. RENDERING PROVIDER ID. #
1									NPI	
2									NPI	
3									NPI	
4									NPI	
5									NPI	
6									NPI	

25. FEDERAL TAX I.D. NUMBER SSN EIN

26. PATIENT'S ACCOUNT NO.

27. ACCEPT ASSIGNMENT? (For govt. claims, see back) YES NO

28. TOTAL CHARGE $

29. AMOUNT PAID $

30. BALANCE DUE $

31. SIGNATURE OF PHYSICIAN OR SUPPLIER INCLUDING DEGREES OR CREDENTIALS (I certify that the statements on the reverse apply to this bill and are made a part thereof.)

SIGNED DATE

32. SERVICE FACILITY LOCATION INFORMATION

a. NPI b.

33. BILLING PROVIDER INFO & PH # ( )

a. NPI b.

PHYSICIAN OR SUPPLIER INFORMATION

SAMPLE

NUCC Instruction Manual available at: www.nucc.org

PLEASE PRINT OR TYPE

APPROVED OMB-0938-0999 FORM CMS-1500 (08-05)

Box 1. Mark (with an X) the appicable box. "Group Health Plan" is the box to use for all forms of health insurance. Check "Other" for work comp or PI claims.

Box 1a. Insured ID Number: This is the insured's policy number, found on their insurance card. As a default and in a rare few cases, the patient's social security number may be used in place of a policy number. Some insurance companies, such as Union carriers, do not issue separate policy numbers but instead use social security numbers. This is *the most important* field on this entire claim. Without being able to identify the patient, the claim cannot even begin to be processed. If this is a claim for a workers compensation case or personal injury, the claim number should be in this field.

2. Patient's Name (last, first format)
3. Patient's Date of Birth and Sex
4. Insured's Name (last, first format) (insured's name may be different from the patient's name if the patient is a spouse or dependent of the insured.)
5. Patient's Address
6. Patient's Relationship to Insured
7. Insured's Address
8. Patient Status (single, married, etc.)
9. Other Insured's Name and information (use only if patient has a secondary insurance policy)
10. Patient's Condition. This field is where you indicate whether the claim is related to a workers compensation or a personal injury (PI) case or other accident. Unless this is due to one of these reasons, all boxes should be checked *no*. This field flags the insurance company to seek reimbursement from the responsible party; they are paying the bill in advance of whomever is responsible. Unless red flags *should* be raised such as the above scenarios, always check *no* to all. Additionally, if a patient was gardening at home, for example, and suffered a low back sprain/strain, you *still* check *no* to accident *unless* someone else's insurance should be paying the bill.
11. This is where the insured's group number goes. It is typically found on the patient's identification card. If it wasn't listed,

hopefully it was asked for during the insurance verification. PI and workers compensation cases do not have group numbers and so you would leave this blank.

11b. If the employer's name is known, list it here. This is not mandatory, just sometimes needed to identify which group the patient belongs to, especially if a group number was not listed in box 11.

11c. Enter the name of the insurance plan or program.

11d. Is there another health benefit plan? Most often, this is checked *no*. If a patient has a secondary insurance, check *yes* and complete box #9.

12. PMS programs will print "signature on file" in this box and should be dated at least on the date of the services being billed on this claim or *prior*.

13. This field should also read "signature on file." For *both* of these fields (12 and 13) that indicate *signature on file*, the signature it refers to is the one where the patient signed an 'assignment of benefits' form. It is kept with the initial paperwork and allows the provider to access and bill the patient's insurance. As long as this form is on file with your office, you can always write "signature on file" in these boxes.

14. This is the date the condition began. If these charges are due to an accident (PI case) or workers compensation injury, the date entered here would be the date of that accident or injury, specifically. For general insurance, enter the date the condition began. Just be careful not to date it *prior* to the date the insurance became effective. For example, if this patient's plan began 1/1/09 and the treatment dates are 2/10/09, don't put an onset date of 12/1/08 in this condition box. It sends the message to the insurance company that this condition existed *prior* to the date the insurance became effective and is therefore *not* their responsibility to pay. This is what is referred to as a pre-existing condition. If this actually is the case, you may need to consider charging the patient cash rates.

15-19. Fields 15-19 are typically left blank.

20. Check *no* for outside lab.

21. Enter the diagnosis codes here. If you have more than the four the claim allows, enter additional codes on line 19. Remember to

enter diagnosis codes to the highest level of specificity; codes have either four or five digits which more specifically identifies the condition. Rarely are they only three digits long. It is a good idea to have a current ICD-9 code book for this reason. You can also find a lot of this information online.

22. Leave blank.
23. Prior Authorization Number: this would primarily pertain to a workers compensation case where one must have prior authorization. If no number was assigned, write what was authorized and by whom (for example, six visits per adjuster—state their name). American Specialty Health will provide an authorization number and it should be listed here. Other than these two instances, nothing needs to be entered in this field.

24a. List the dates of service, each line is for one date of service. For example, a date of service of 2/11/09 would be written *from* 02112009 *to* 02112009.

24b. Place of service is always listed as '11' if services were provided in an office environment. '12' would be listed for services performed in a patient's home. For other places of service, see our website for a complete list.

24c. Leave blank.

24d. List the current procedure terminology (CPT) code for the appropriate service being billed. If there is a modifier, you would list a modifier next to the CPT code. To know if you need a modifier, see the modifier section of this book. Remember, if you are using an Evaluation & Management (E & M) code at the same visit as a procedure, it needs to have a -25 modifier.

24e. This field connects the diagnosis code and the CPT code. For example, if the following diagnoses are in field 1 (of box 21) 723.1 (cervical pain) and in field 2: 724.1 (thoracic pain), when the new patient exam code of 99203 is entered, on that corresponding line in box 24e would be 1, 2, meaning that the exam was for both the cervical and thoracic pain. If therapies are billed with the treatment, perhaps you might list a 97026 for infrared, next to it, in box 24e, the diagnosis codes need to be entered. Do not use commas or punctuation.

24f. This is the charge for the service being billed. *The full fee for each code as listed in your fee schedule should be entered.* If you know that the fee(s) will get discounted based on contractual reductions, do *not* bill those reduced amounts, instead leave the fees and let the insurance company reduce them.

24g. Days or units pertain to the number of units of that particular service being billed. Initial acupuncture is a single unit procedure so it would always have a '1' in the unit box. A service such as 97140 or 97124 for bodywork, however, could have more than 1 unit since it is a time based procedure and is therefore billed in 15-minute increments (or the better part thereof). So, if you performed 23 minutes of manual therapy or massage to the patient, you would enter a '2' in box 24g. A CPT code book will list each CPT code and will indicate if it is a time based procedure or not. This information will help determine how many units of a procedure should be billed based on the time spent performing the procedure.

24h-i. Leave blank.

24j. This field must be completed with your NPI number.

25. If you have a tax identification number, it should be entered here. If you are using only your social security number (though this is not a good idea), list it here. Put an X in the box your number corresponds to.

26. The Patient Account Number field is exclusively for your benefit. The insurance typically would list this account number on the explanation of benefits (EOBs) they send, so this number is purely for identification purposes. If this doesn't matter and you can identify the patient by name, then this field does not need to be completed.

27. The 'Accept Assignment' field is *extremely important*. If this box is marked '*no*' then the payment will be sent to the patient. If this box is marked '*yes*' then the payment will be sent to the provider (you).

28. This is a sum of the above charges billed.

Box 29 and 30 do not need to be completed.

31. You do *not* need to sign each claim. If you have a PMS that generates the claims for you, it will simply print your name in the

field. If you were manually completing this form, there is no need to do more than print your name.

32. This box does not need to be completed if the address is the same as box #33.
33. List your clinic name or practitioner name along with the telephone number and address of the clinic. Payments will be sent to this address.

33a. You will again list your NPI here.

Claim forms are relatively inexpensive and can be purchased via many companies; this author uses Rx data systems but you can also conduct a search on-line to do a price comparison.

Case Study

While preparing to bill a VA patient's first visit, I realize that there is no authorization information in the computer, therefore no authorization number will populate (as needed) onto the claim form. Thankfully, the receptionist had remembered to get a copy of the authorization so that the information could be input, which allowed the CMS 1500 to be completed properly and submitted for payment.

Online Submission of Claims

In addition to completing and submitting a CMS 1500 form, you can also submit your claim information online directly to the insurance company. Many insurances now accept claims electronically either by bulk download or simply by entering your claims individually, online. Once you have gained access to an insurance company's online system, you can submit claims online as well as track their payment status. You should register to become a user of this feature at each insurance company's website. Remember that you can also use this access to check eligibility and verify benefits in some cases. Although this information is typically not thorough enough to rely upon, it can provide a double check or piece of the puzzle if eligibility is in question.

Claims follow-up

After you submit your claims, the follow-up phase begins. Hopefully the follow-up will consist of posting payments and writing off balances (see note below). If, however, you receive claim denials, they must be responded to.

Be aware that each insurance company has different "time frames for submission" and you must follow-up on outstanding claims within these time frames so they are not flat out denied. Time frames for submission should be asked about during the insurance verification.

That being said, let's begin the process. First of all, if a claim is paid, you will need to apply the payment appropriately to the patient's account in the practice management software (PMS) or however you are tracking patient payments and balances. If there is a balance owed by the patient, the bill should immediately be sent to the patient. When billing the patient, always make it clear what the balance is for, have a due date for the payment and, unless you have a ton of these, handwrite "thank you" on the statement. You may also want to include a quick explanation as to why there is a balance to avoid a phone call from the patient and include a copy of the explanation of benefits (EOB) as a

Note

Writing off balances is the difference between what you charged and what you collected or can expect to collect. For example, I may charge Acupuncture (97810) at $60 to American Specialty Health (ASH). Under contract, I have agreed to accept $40/visit which includes both the amount ASH will pay and what the patient is responsible for. So, ASH will process the $60 charge at $40 then say the patient has a responsibility of $14 and so they will pay $26. I now need to post the payment of $26 from ASH, hopefully having already collected the $14 patient portion, and then write off the other $20 that I will not receive. You should always charge your established fee schedule amounts to insurance companies. Let each payor reduce your charges based on your contracts with them. Not only is it the law (to have one fee schedule), this establishes our usual and customary rates in our industry and you don't ever want to shortchange yourself in case more starts being paid.

quick reference. It is also helpful to highlight the pertinent information on that EOB so that the patient easily understands the balance they are responsible for.

If the claim was not paid, you need to determine why. Learning to read EOBs can take some time. They look more intimidating than they really are so one must slowly and methodically approach them. The first column usually consists of the total billed amount. The next column typically shows the "allowed amount" or the allowed amount by the insurance if you are a contracted provider. This is the amount that you have agreed to accept by being a contracted provider. It will, more than likely, be reduced from what was originally billed. The next column should list the explanation code(s) for the reduction. A usual explanation would be that it is your provider discount. Other explanations can include the service not being covered or sometimes included in the cost of another procedure, etc. This explanation may or may not be accurate. This is a common mistake: codes are denied citing they are combined with another procedure. More on this later. The next column(s) relate to deductibles, co-pays, or co-insurance amounts owed by the patient. The last column is always what amount was paid to the provider. If the claim or certain charges were not paid, you need to conclude why they weren't, from this you need to determine the best way to dispute it. If it was a simple mathematical error (for example, the insurance is saying visits exceeded the benefit but you believe this to be untrue), you can simply call the insurance company and inquire. Usually they will send the claim back through for reprocessing and you wait (and hope) they fix the problem and pay you. This may or may not resolve the claim. If not, you may need to call the insurance company again and play the back and forth game until you get resolution.

Sometimes claims will be denied because they require medical justification. If so, you may need to submit chart notes and/or medical reports. Make sure that you review your notes prior to submission for accuracy since once you submit your notes, you cannot retract them. It is just good practice to do a review of any information you send prior to submission, in all cases. If you are unable to get satisfactory claim resolution, you can call the insurance company and ask to speak to a supervisor. Sometimes this can be helpful. You can try writing a letter to the insurance company, stating your issue and why you are appealing the decision made by them. This is, frustratingly, not very effective in most cases. You would swear these letters go straight into a shredder and so you do always have the option of sending it certified with a return receipt. If all of your attempts fail and you are completely fed up, you can file a written, formal complaint to the insurance commissioner. If it comes to this, you will want to submit all communications to support your efforts to resolve your issue up until that point. Insurance commissioner complaints should not be done often and only when a significant issue is present, probably something that keeps recurring, and is in need of adjudication.

You should document all efforts made to resolve any claim. Many times, when following up on a claim, this author will have to review all previous notes in order to explain what has transpired to date, to the next customer service representative currently trying to help resolve the claim. It is very helpful to have this information in chronological order, easily accessible, and succinct when re-explaining and/or documenting the issue.

Case Study

After not receiving payment for 60 days on a work comp claim, I happily pulled the written authorization, copied it and sent it in with the claim and tracer. Payment was received two weeks later.

When posting insurance payments to a patient's account, do you look at other bills that are outstanding in that patient's account? What do you send with bills that need to be resubmitted? At what point do you call the insurance company instead of resubmitting?

EOB Samples

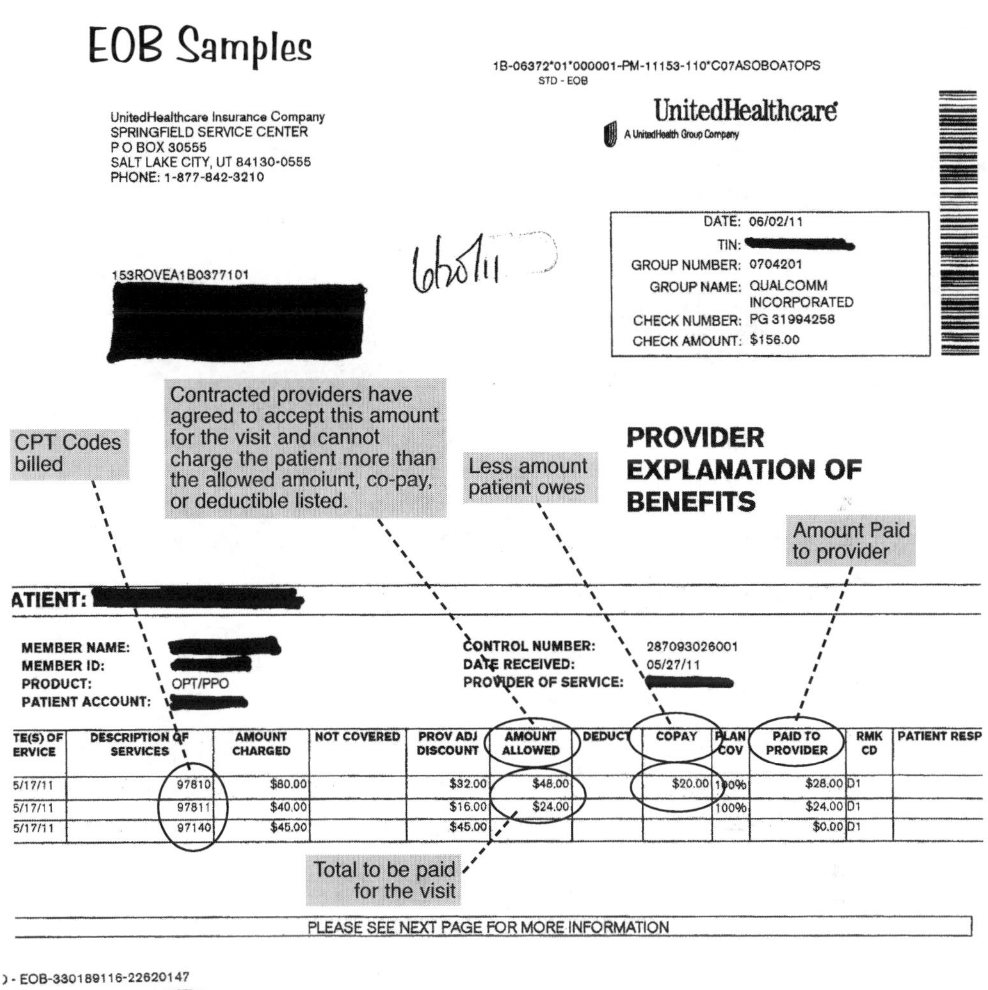

1B-06372*01*000001-PM-11153-110*C07ASOBOATOPS
STD - EOB

UnitedHealthcare Insurance Company
SPRINGFIELD SERVICE CENTER
P O BOX 30555
SALT LAKE CITY, UT 84130-0555
PHONE: 1-877-842-3210

UnitedHealthcare
A UnitedHealth Group Company

DATE: 06/02/11
TIN:
GROUP NUMBER: 0704201
GROUP NAME: QUALCOMM INCORPORATED
CHECK NUMBER: PG 31994258
CHECK AMOUNT: $156.00

153ROVEA1B0377101

PROVIDER EXPLANATION OF BENEFITS

ATIENT:

MEMBER NAME:
MEMBER ID:
PRODUCT: OPT/PPO
PATIENT ACCOUNT:

CONTROL NUMBER: 287093026001
DATE RECEIVED: 05/27/11
PROVIDER OF SERVICE:

TE(S) OF ERVICE	DESCRIPTION OF SERVICES	AMOUNT CHARGED	NOT COVERED	PROV ADJ DISCOUNT	AMOUNT ALLOWED	DEDUCT	COPAY	PLAN COV	PAID TO PROVIDER	RMK CD	PATIENT RESP
5/17/11	97810	$80.00		$32.00	$48.00		$20.00	100%	$28.00	D1	
5/17/11	97811	$40.00		$16.00	$24.00			100%	$24.00	D1	
5/17/11	97140	$45.00		$45.00					$0.00	D1	

PLEASE SEE NEXT PAGE FOR MORE INFORMATION

) - EOB-330189116-22620147
PATIENT ACCOUNT:

TE(S) OF ERVICE	DESCRIPTION OF SERVICES	AMOUNT CHARGED	NOT COVERED	PROV ADJ DISCOUNT	AMOUNT ALLOWED	DEDUCT	COPAY	PLAN COV	PAID TO PROVIDER	RMK CD	PATIENT RESP
5/14/11	97810	$80.00		$32.00	$48.00		$20.00	100%	$28.00	D1	
5/14/11	97811	$40.00		$16.00	$24.00			100%	$24.00	D1	
5/14/11	97140	$45.00		$45.00					$0.00	D1	
5/14/11	97026	$20.00		$20.00					$0.00	D1	
5/14/11	97010	$10.00	$10.00	$10.00					$0.00	4	
CONTROL # 287093026102 SUBTOTAL:		$195.00	$10.00	$123.00	$72.00		$20.00		$52.00	#	$20.00
						TOTAL PAYABLE TO PROVIDER			$156.00		

MARKS:

THANK YOU FOR USING A NETWORK PHYSICIAN OR OTHER HEALTH CARE PROFESSIONAL. WE HAVE APPLIED THE CONTRACTED FEE. THE PATIENT IS NOT RESPONSIBLE FOR THE DIFFERENCE BETWEEN THE AMOUNT CHARGED BY THE PHYSICIAN OR HEALTH CARE PROFESSIONAL AND THE AMOUNT ALLOWED BY THE CONTRACT, EXCEPT IN SITUATIONS WHERE THERE IS AN ANNUAL BENEFIT MAXIMUM FOR THIS SERVICE. THE PATIENT IS ALSO RESPONSIBLE FOR ANY COPAY, DEDUCTIBLE AND COINSURANCE AMOUNTS.

THIS IS NOT A SEPARATELY REIMBURSABLE SERVICE OR SUPPLY.

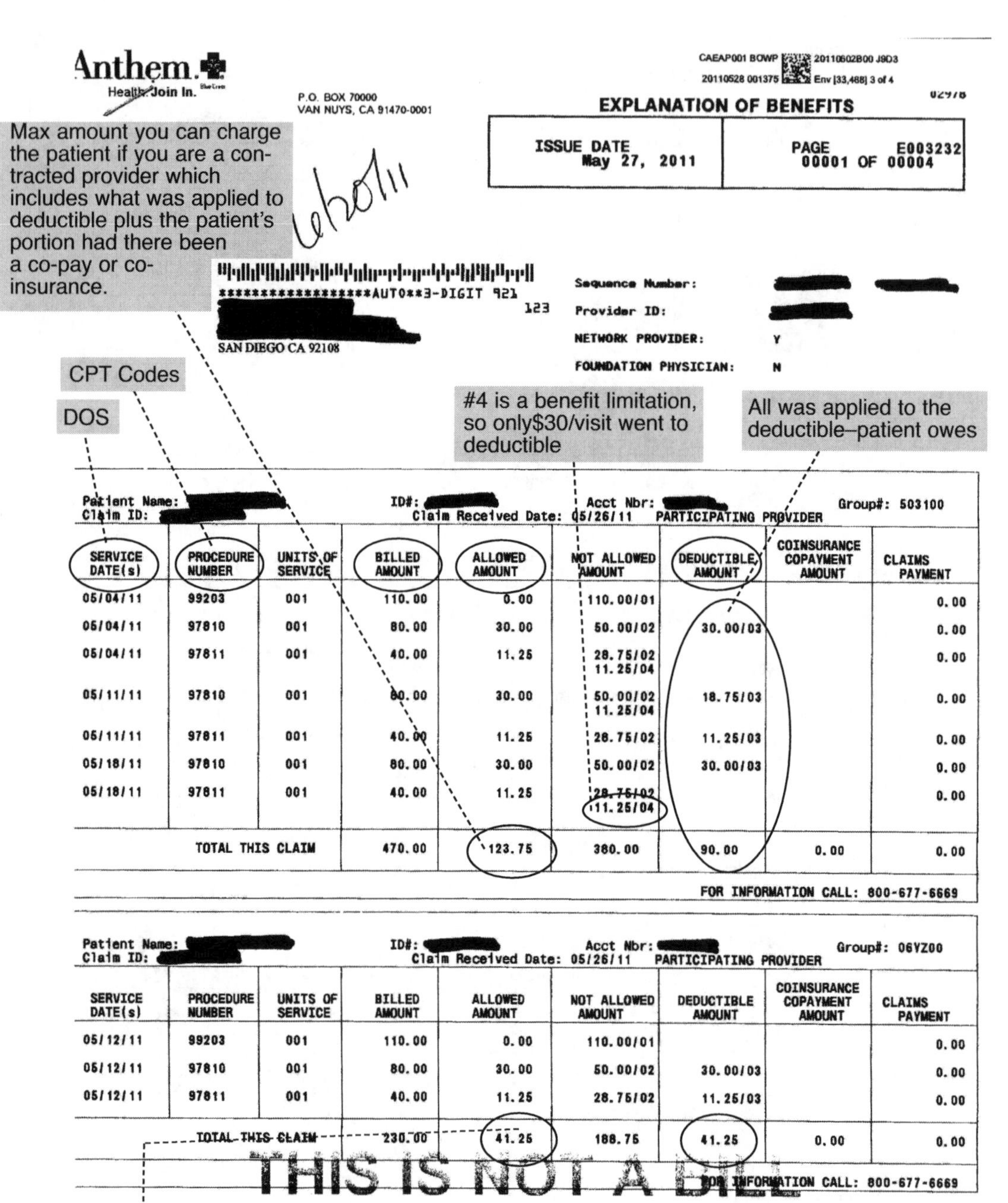

Anthem. Health Join In.

P.O. BOX 70000
VAN NUYS, CA 91470-0001

CAEAP001 BOWP 20110602B00 J9D3
20110528 001375 Env [33,488] 3 of 4

EXPLANATION OF BENEFITS

ISSUE DATE	PAGE E003232
May 27, 2011	00001 OF 00004

******************AUTO**3-DIGIT 921
123
SAN DIEGO CA 92108

Sequence Number:
Provider ID:
NETWORK PROVIDER: Y
FOUNDATION PHYSICIAN: N

Patient Name: ID#: Acct Nbr: Group#: 503100
Claim ID: Claim Received Date: 05/26/11 PARTICIPATING PROVIDER

SERVICE DATE(s)	PROCEDURE NUMBER	UNITS OF SERVICE	BILLED AMOUNT	ALLOWED AMOUNT	NOT ALLOWED AMOUNT	DEDUCTIBLE AMOUNT	COINSURANCE COPAYMENT AMOUNT	CLAIMS PAYMENT
05/04/11	99203	001	110.00	0.00	110.00/01			0.00
05/04/11	97810	001	80.00	30.00	50.00/02	30.00/03		0.00
05/04/11	97811	001	40.00	11.25	28.75/02 11.25/04			0.00
05/11/11	97810	001	80.00	30.00	50.00/02 11.25/04	18.75/03		0.00
05/11/11	97811	001	40.00	11.25	28.75/02	11.25/03		0.00
05/18/11	97810	001	80.00	30.00	50.00/02	30.00/03		0.00
05/18/11	97811	001	40.00	11.25	28.75/02 11.25/04			0.00
	TOTAL THIS CLAIM		470.00	123.75	380.00	90.00	0.00	0.00

FOR INFORMATION CALL: 800-677-6669

Patient Name: ID#: Acct Nbr: Group#: 06VZ00
Claim ID: Claim Received Date: 05/26/11 PARTICIPATING PROVIDER

SERVICE DATE(s)	PROCEDURE NUMBER	UNITS OF SERVICE	BILLED AMOUNT	ALLOWED AMOUNT	NOT ALLOWED AMOUNT	DEDUCTIBLE AMOUNT	COINSURANCE COPAYMENT AMOUNT	CLAIMS PAYMENT
05/12/11	99203	001	110.00	0.00	110.00/01			0.00
05/12/11	97810	001	80.00	30.00	50.00/02	30.00/03		0.00
05/12/11	97811	001	40.00	11.25	28.75/02	11.25/03		0.00
	TOTAL THIS CLAIM		230.00	41.25	188.75	41.25	0.00	0.00

THIS IS NOT A BILL

FOR INFORMATION CALL: 800-677-6669

All of the allowed amount went towards deductible and is owed by the patient. This is more typical, unlike other patient above.

Anthem Blue Cross is the trade name of Blue Cross of California. Independent licensee of the Blue Cross Association. ® ANTHEM is a registered trademark of Anthem Insurance Companies, Inc. The Blue Cross names and symbols are registered marks of the Blue Cross Association.

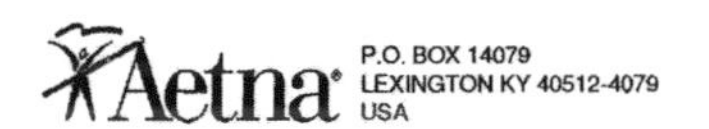

P.O. BOX 14079
LEXINGTON KY 40512-4079
USA

EXPLANATION OF BENEFITS

Please Retain for Future Referenc

Check No: 08325-07900212
Page 2 of 2 (1)

Date Printed:	06/01/2011
Tax Identification Number:	XXXXXXXX9116

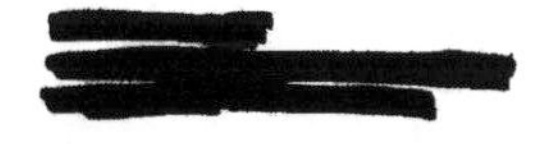

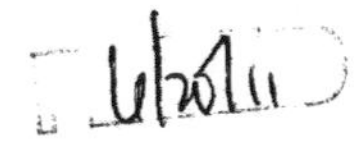

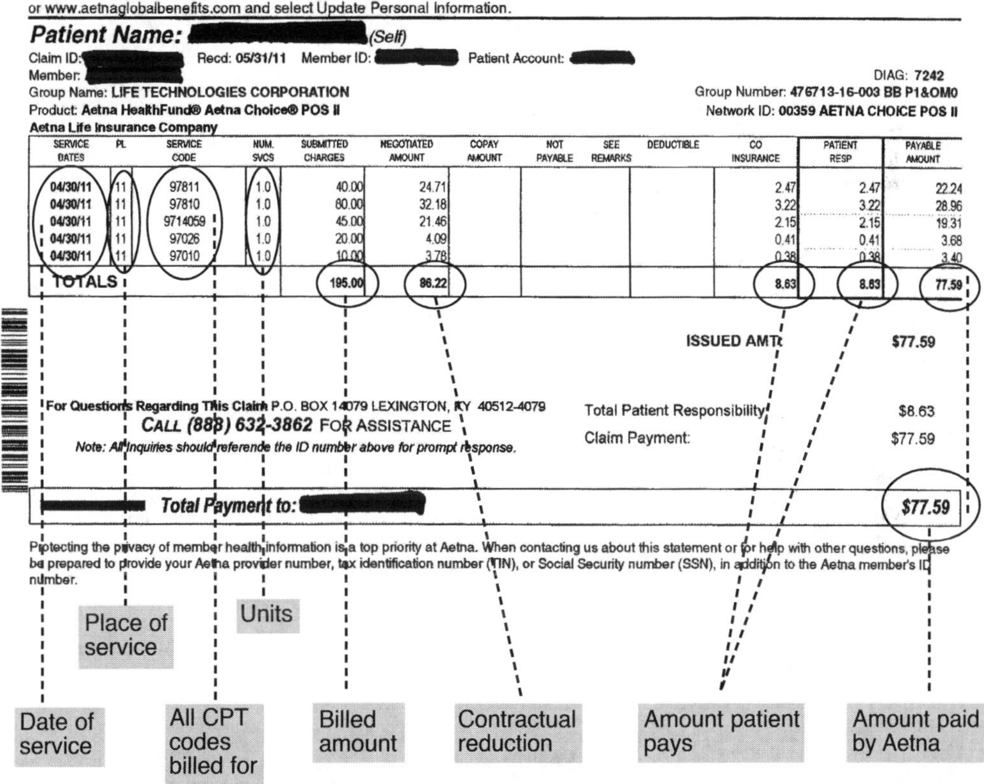

Notes:

Update your address, telephone number, email address and/or NPI information by visiting www.aetna.com/provweb/, www.aetnadental.com or www.aetnaglobalbenefits.com and select Update Personal Information.

Patient Name: *(Self)*

Claim ID: Recd: **05/31/11** Member ID: Patient Account:

Member: DIAG: **7242**

Group Name: **LIFE TECHNOLOGIES CORPORATION** Group Number: **476713-16-003 BB P1&OM0**

Product: **Aetna HealthFund® Aetna Choice® POS II** Network ID: **00359 AETNA CHOICE POS II**

Aetna Life Insurance Company

SERVICE DATES	PL	SERVICE CODE	NUM. SVCS	SUBMITTED CHARGES	NEGOTIATED AMOUNT	COPAY AMOUNT	NOT PAYABLE	SEE REMARKS	DEDUCTIBLE	CO INSURANCE	PATIENT RESP	PAYABLE AMOUNT
04/30/11	11	97811	1.0	40.00	24.71					2.47	2.47	22.24
04/30/11	11	97810	1.0	80.00	32.18					3.22	3.22	28.96
04/30/11	11	9714059	1.0	45.00	21.46					2.15	2.15	19.31
04/30/11	11	97026	1.0	20.00	4.09					0.41	0.41	3.68
04/30/11	11	97010	1.0	10.00	3.78					0.38	0.38	3.40
TOTALS				**195.00**	**86.22**					**8.63**	**8.63**	**77.59**

ISSUED AMT **$77.59**

For Questions Regarding This Claim P.O. BOX 14079 LEXINGTON, KY 40512-4079
CALL (888) 632-3862 FOR ASSISTANCE
Note: All Inquiries should reference the ID number above for prompt response.

Total Patient Responsibility: $8.63
Claim Payment: $77.59

Total Payment to: ***$77.59***

Protecting the privacy of member health information is a top priority at Aetna. When contacting us about this statement or for help with other questions, please be prepared to provide your Aetna provider number, tax identification number (TIN), or Social Security number (SSN), in addition to the Aetna member's ID number.

Workers' Comp EOB Sample

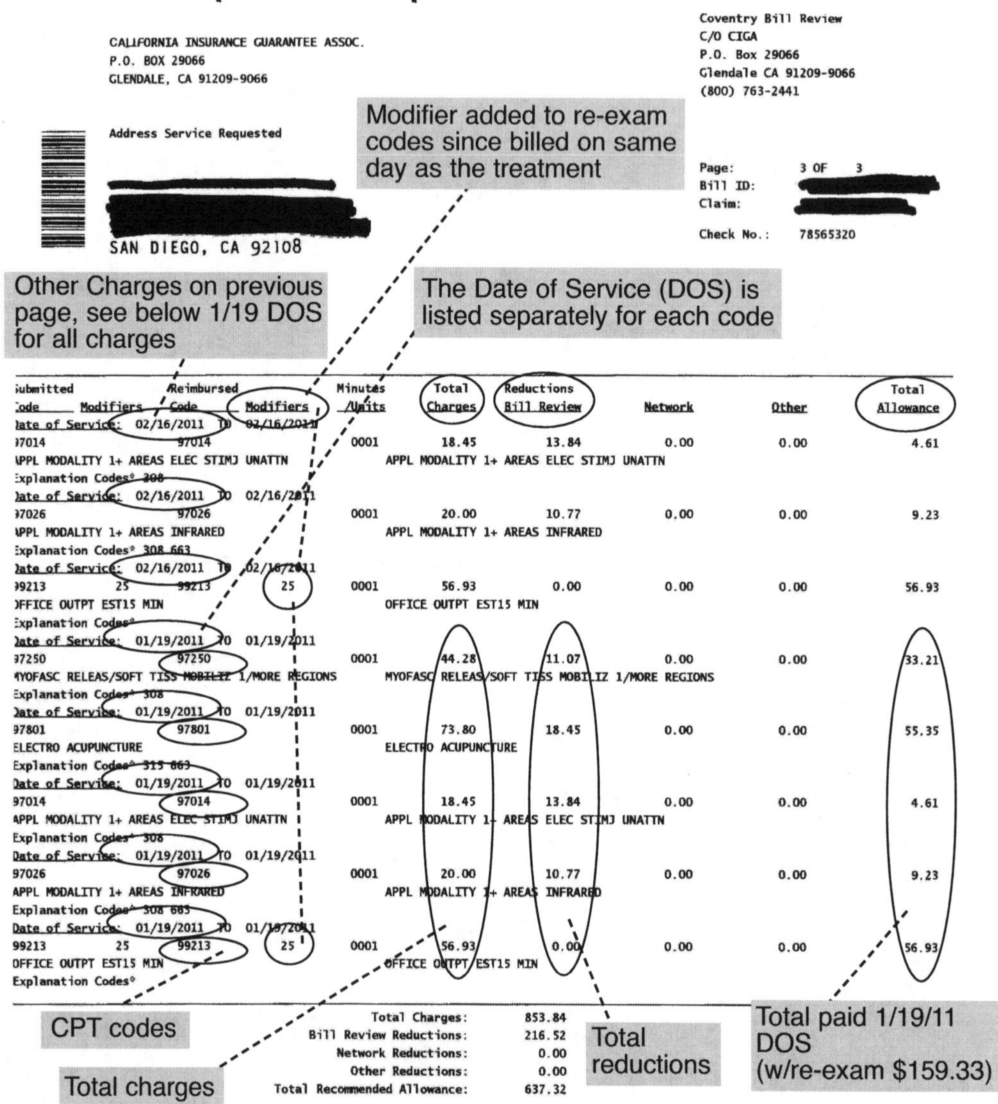

CALIFORNIA INSURANCE GUARANTEE ASSOC.
P.O. BOX 29066
GLENDALE, CA 91209-9066

Coventry Bill Review
C/O CIGA
P.O. Box 29066
Glendale CA 91209-9066
(800) 763-2441

Address Service Requested

SAN DIEGO, CA 92108

Page: 3 OF 3
Bill ID:
Claim:

Check No.: 78565320

Submitted Code	Modifiers	Reimbursed Code	Modifiers	Minutes /Units	Total Charges	Reductions Bill Review	Network	Other	Total Allowance
Date of Service: 02/16/2011 TO 02/16/2011									
97014		97014		0001	18.45	13.84	0.00	0.00	4.61
APPL MODALITY 1+ AREAS ELEC STIMJ UNATTN		APPL MODALITY 1+ AREAS ELEC STIMJ UNATTN							
Explanation Codes* 308									
Date of Service: 02/16/2011 TO 02/16/2011									
97026		97026		0001	20.00	10.77	0.00	0.00	9.23
APPL MODALITY 1+ AREAS INFRARED		APPL MODALITY 1+ AREAS INFRARED							
Explanation Codes* 308 663									
Date of Service: 02/16/2011 TO 02/16/2011									
99213	25	99213	25	0001	56.93	0.00	0.00	0.00	56.93
OFFICE OUTPT EST15 MIN		OFFICE OUTPT EST15 MIN							
Explanation Codes*									
Date of Service: 01/19/2011 TO 01/19/2011									
97250		97250		0001	44.28	11.07	0.00	0.00	33.21
MYOFASC RELEAS/SOFT TISS MOBILIZ 1/MORE REGIONS		MYOFASC RELEAS/SOFT TISS MOBILIZ 1/MORE REGIONS							
Explanation Codes* 308									
Date of Service: 01/19/2011 TO 01/19/2011									
97801		97801		0001	73.80	18.45	0.00	0.00	55.35
ELECTRO ACUPUNCTURE		ELECTRO ACUPUNCTURE							
Explanation Codes* 315 663									
Date of Service: 01/19/2011 TO 01/19/2011									
97014		97014		0001	18.45	13.84	0.00	0.00	4.61
APPL MODALITY 1+ AREAS ELEC STIMJ UNATTN		APPL MODALITY 1+ AREAS ELEC STIMJ UNATTN							
Explanation Codes* 308									
Date of Service: 01/19/2011 TO 01/19/2011									
97026		97026		0001	20.00	10.77	0.00	0.00	9.23
APPL MODALITY 1+ AREAS INFRARED		APPL MODALITY 1+ AREAS INFRARED							
Explanation Codes* 308 663									
Date of Service: 01/19/2011 TO 01/19/2011									
99213	25	99213	25	0001	56.93	0.00	0.00	0.00	56.93
OFFICE OUTPT EST15 MIN		OFFICE OUTPT EST15 MIN							
Explanation Codes*									

Total Charges:	853.84
Bill Review Reductions:	216.52
Network Reductions:	0.00
Other Reductions:	0.00
Total Recommended Allowance:	637.32

308 THE REIMBURSEMENT HAS BEEN CALCULATED ACCORDING TO THE PHYSICAL MEDICINE MULTIPLE PROCEDURE GUIDELINES.
315 SINCE PHYSICAL MEDICINE INCLUDES EVALUATION OF THE PATIENT, REIMBURSEMENT WILL BE REDUCED FOR AN OFFICE VISIT BILLED ON THE SAME DAY AS PHYSICIAL MEDICINE.
663 REIMBURSEMENT HAS BEEN CALCULATED ACCORDING TO STATE FEE SCHEDULE GUIDELINES

Unless otherwise noted, all reductions are in accordance with the medical fee schedule as per the rules and regulations authorized by California Labor Code Section 4603.5 and 5307.1. The treating physician or authorized provider may adjudicate the issue of the contested charges before the Workers' Compensation Appeals Board.
If you have any questions regarding this analysis, please call Coventry at (800) 763-2441 or send your bill and this analysis with your request to: CIGA, P.O. Box 29066, Glendale CA 91209-9066.

Cigna EOB Sample

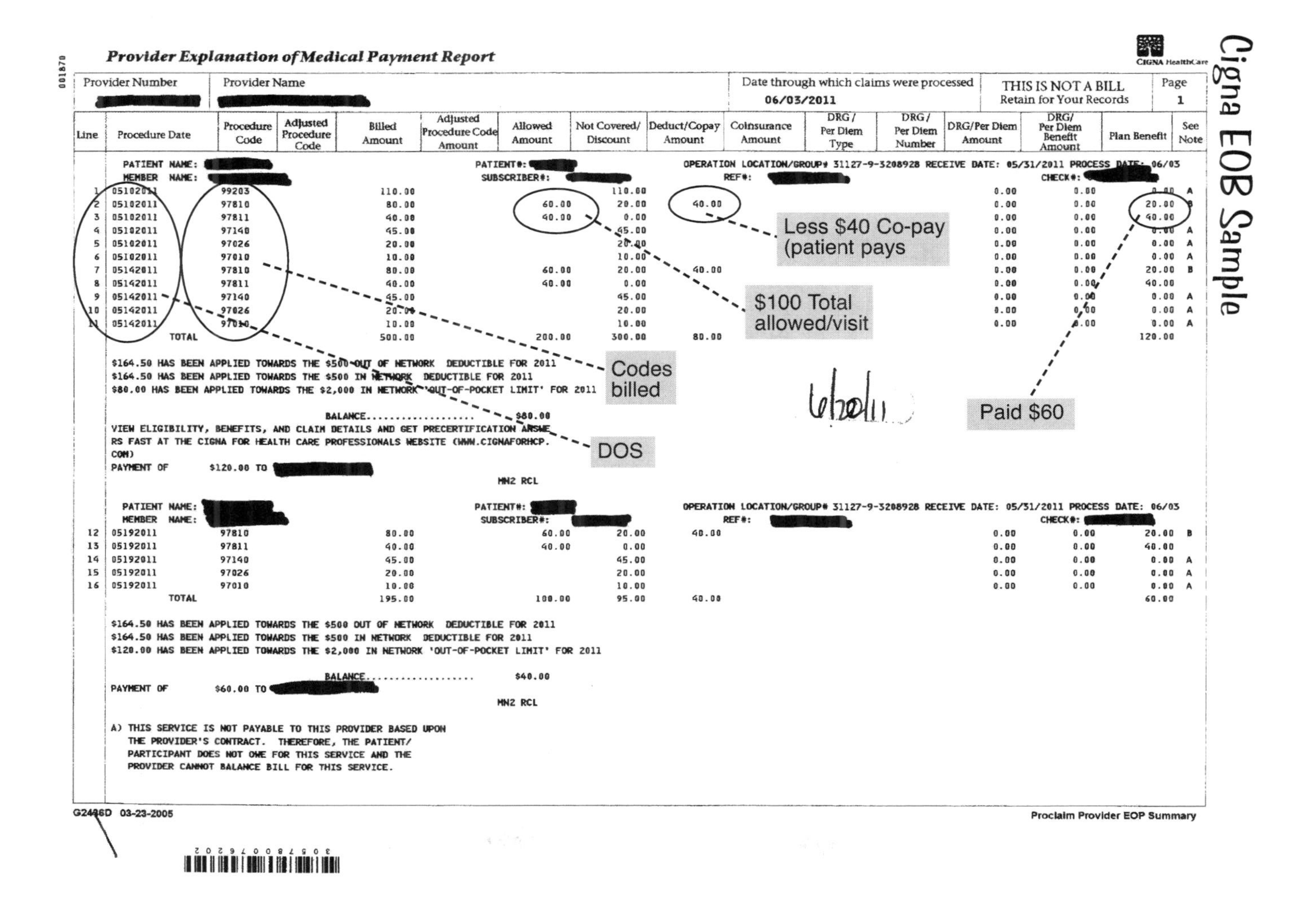

CIGNA HealthCare

Provider Explanation of Medical Payment Report

Provider Number	Provider Name	Date through which claims were processed	THIS IS NOT A BILL	Page
		06/03/2011	Retain for Your Records	1

PATIENT NAME: PATIENT#: OPERATION LOCATION/GROUP# 31127-9-3208928 RECEIVE DATE: 05/31/2011 PROCESS DATE: 06/03

MEMBER NAME: SUBSCRIBER#: REF#: CHECK#:

Line	Procedure Date	Procedure Code	Adjusted Procedure Code	Billed Amount	Adjusted Procedure Code Amount	Allowed Amount	Not Covered/ Discount	Deduct/Copay Amount	Coinsurance Amount	DRG/ Per Diem Type	DRG/ Per Diem Number	DRG/Per Diem Amount	DRG/ Per Diem Benefit Amount	Plan Benefit	See Note
1	05102011	99203		110.00			110.00					0.00	0.00	0.00	A
2	05102011	97810		80.00		60.00	20.00	40.00				0.00	0.00	20.00	B
3	05102011	97811		40.00		40.00	0.00					0.00	0.00	40.00	
4	05102011	97140		45.00			45.00					0.00	0.00	0.00	A
5	05102011	97026		20.00			20.00					0.00	0.00	0.00	A
6	05102011	97010		10.00			10.00					0.00	0.00	0.00	A
7	05142011	97810		80.00		60.00	20.00	40.00				0.00	0.00	20.00	B
8	05142011	97811		40.00		40.00	0.00					0.00	0.00	40.00	
9	05142011	97140		45.00			45.00					0.00	0.00	0.00	A
10	05142011	97026		20.00			20.00					0.00	0.00	0.00	A
11	05142011	97010		10.00			10.00					0.00	0.00	0.00	A
	TOTAL			500.00		200.00	300.00	80.00						120.00	

$164.50 HAS BEEN APPLIED TOWARDS THE $500 OUT OF NETWORK DEDUCTIBLE FOR 2011
$164.50 HAS BEEN APPLIED TOWARDS THE $500 IN NETWORK DEDUCTIBLE FOR 2011
$80.00 HAS BEEN APPLIED TOWARDS THE $2,000 IN NETWORK 'OUT-OF-POCKET LIMIT' FOR 2011

BALANCE.................. $80.00

VIEW ELIGIBILITY, BENEFITS, AND CLAIM DETAILS AND GET PRECERTIFICATION ANSWERS FAST AT THE CIGNA FOR HEALTH CARE PROFESSIONALS WEBSITE (WWW.CIGNAFORHCP.COM)

PAYMENT OF $120.00 TO

MN2 RCL

PATIENT NAME: PATIENT#: OPERATION LOCATION/GROUP# 31127-9-3208928 RECEIVE DATE: 05/31/2011 PROCESS DATE: 06/03

MEMBER NAME: SUBSCRIBER#: REF#: CHECK#:

Line	Procedure Date	Procedure Code	Adjusted Procedure Code	Billed Amount	Adjusted Procedure Code Amount	Allowed Amount	Not Covered/ Discount	Deduct/Copay Amount	Coinsurance Amount	DRG/ Per Diem Type	DRG/ Per Diem Number	DRG/Per Diem Amount	DRG/ Per Diem Benefit Amount	Plan Benefit	See Note
12	05192011	97810		80.00		60.00	20.00	40.00				0.00	0.00	20.00	B
13	05192011	97811		40.00		40.00	0.00					0.00	0.00	40.00	
14	05192011	97140		45.00			45.00					0.00	0.00	0.00	A
15	05192011	97026		20.00			20.00					0.00	0.00	0.00	A
16	05192011	97010		10.00			10.00					0.00	0.00	0.00	A
	TOTAL			195.00		100.00	95.00	40.00						60.00	

$164.50 HAS BEEN APPLIED TOWARDS THE $500 OUT OF NETWORK DEDUCTIBLE FOR 2011
$164.50 HAS BEEN APPLIED TOWARDS THE $500 IN NETWORK DEDUCTIBLE FOR 2011
$120.00 HAS BEEN APPLIED TOWARDS THE $2,000 IN NETWORK 'OUT-OF-POCKET LIMIT' FOR 2011

BALANCE.................. $40.00

PAYMENT OF $60.00 TO

MN2 RCL

A) THIS SERVICE IS NOT PAYABLE TO THIS PROVIDER BASED UPON THE PROVIDER'S CONTRACT. THEREFORE, THE PATIENT/PARTICIPANT DOES NOT OWE FOR THIS SERVICE AND THE PROVIDER CANNOT BALANCE BILL FOR THIS SERVICE.

G2486D 03-23-2005

Proclaim Provider EOP Summary

Daily, Weekly, Monthly, and Annual Insurance Procedures

7

Checklist for Chapter 7:

- Do end-of-day balancing
  - Keep track of daily statistics
- Do weekly procedures
  - Post all received payments
  - Generate bills
  - Resubmit claims, possibly with a tracer for any outstanding claims
- Do monthly procedures
  - Run reports from the practice management software
  - Keep track of monthly statistics
  - Follow up on receivables
- Do annual procedures
  - Re-verify every patient's insurance (when they come and see you)
  - Summarize annual statistics

One should plan on billing and following up on accounts receivables on a regular basis and set a schedule accordingly as an office policy. Although one can bill daily, this can be a bit cumbersome if an office is very busy. Once per week is a good practice and what this author recommends. Twice per month is the maximum one should wait to bill. Whatever billing frequency you establish as your office policy, maintain it for consistent cash flow. For purposes of describing the following schedule, the assumption will be billing is being done weekly with follow-up being done monthly.

Daily tasks

There is nothing specific to insurance billing that must be done at the end of each day. It is very important to follow the end-of-day balancing procedures in order to ensure all patient visits have been entered into the practice management software system and are ready for billing. This means ensuring that all insurance verifications have been completed, policy info entered, diagnosis for billing, correct charges, etc. The authors recommend that you keep basic statistics to track office progress. Daily statistics would report on such things as: number of visits, total charges, total received, new patients, etc.

Case Study

Are you tracking your daily statistics? Do you have balancing procedures in place to ensure the accuracy of the information and money collected each day?

While reviewing yesterday's day sheet (report of all entries into the medical software system used in the office), I see that the amount of cash received on the report is $200, but what is in the accompanying envelope is $225. After reviewing the cash log that the front desk keeps of all cash received (for this very reason) it is realized that a patient's co-pay was collected but not entered. Subsequently, the co-pay was entered, the day sheet was reprinted and now reflected the $225 in cash that was actually received. Thanks to proper balancing procedures, the patient didn't get a bill for the outstanding $25 that they already paid.

The New Year is a good time to recap your year's statistics; total new patients, total patients seen, total charges, total received, etc. This information helps you to make decisions about where to focus your practice in the coming year. How many more new patients did you have this past year compared to the prior? Is your practice growing? Did you try different marketing tactics that may have positively or negatively impacted your practice? Some basic statistics can be very helpful to help paint a picture of your overall business health.

Weekly tasks

Payer payments should be posted to individual patient bills *prior* to generating any new billing. This is a good time to look back on any outstanding bills and inquire into any unpaid bills. This can start with a resubmission of the claim, possibly with a **tracer** attached (see box below), or making a call to the insurance company to check status. Next, prepare your current billing ensuring that any missing information has been inputted such as diagnosis codes and patient identification numbers. Generate and send your bills following the procedure for your practice management software.

Sample tracer letter

Many medical management software programs will generate tracers for you. They will automatically input most of the data listed that was derived from the claim the system generated. If the billing program you use does not offer the feature, I would create a modifiable template to send with subsequent billings that you are following up on. (See the following page for a sample.)

Monthly tasks

Run reports from your practice management software showing outstanding patient balances. This author likes to break them down by insurance, work comp and personal injury. Choose the best report(s) to work from and begin researching outstanding claims and work on collecting on them. These lists should be kept in a billing binder separated by case type to keep it organized. Each subsequent month's report should go on top of the old to, at a glance, track progress. More on this under accounts receivables follow-up below. As with daily statistics, one should keep monthly statistics that summarizes the data from the daily statistics so that you can compare month-to-month practice data. Monthly statistics should also address insurance billing and receivables

INSURANCE TRACER SAMPLE
December 28, 2010

Doctor: Smith & Jones Acupuncture
1234 Main Street
San Diego, CA 92108
619-555-1212
ID No.: 12345678

Patient: John Doe
9876 Washington Blvd
San Diego, CA 92115
DOB: 08/08/1988
Acct No.: 978654

Insured: John Doe
Date of illness or injury: 01/01/10
Employer:
Group No:
Claim/Certificate No.: AB123456
Diagnosis:722.10 Displacement Of Lumbar Intervertebral Disc W/O Myelopathy
847.1 Thoracic Sprain/Strain
847.0 Cervical sprain/strain
Date Billed: 02/27/10
Billed to: State Compensation Fund
Billing Period: 02/26/10 - 02/26/10
Amt. Billed: $150.00
___ Copy of bill attached

It has come to our attention that the above mentioned claim for our Patient / your insured has not been satisfied. In order to satisfactorily adjust our records, we request that you supply the following information on the above named Patient / insured:

Claim Pending Because:
Payment of Claim in Process:
Payment Made on Claim. Date:
To Whom:
Claim Denied: (Reason)
Patient Notified: Yes( ) No( )
Remarks:

Thank you in advance for your prompt assistance in this matter.

To: State Insurance Fund
4567 Day Street
San Diego CA 92108

totals. It is good practice to establish office statistics so you have hard data to compare month to month. This way you will know if your collections are up or down or right in line with normal based on total charges, patient visit totals, etc.

Accounts receivables follow-up

One should be aware of the timely filing requirements of each insurance carrier; some are 90 days, 180 days or even one year. Workers comp and personal injury cases have time frames dictated by the length of the case. It is important to know how much time you have to collect on accounts. This is also why it is a good idea to submit electronically if you can, so reports can be printed proving your claims were submitted in a timely fashion. This proof is helpful when insurance companies come back and say you did not file your claims within the allowed time frame and therefore your claim is denied. Having proof to be able to fight this issue is liberating. American Specialty Health (ASH) issues log numbers that coincide with any issue you may be having. Keep these numbers as it proves you started working on your issue within the appropriate time frame, even if it takes longer to resolve. More on ASH filing requirements in the section that discusses ASH specifically. Similarly, one should always request reference numbers at the conclusion of any phone call to an insurance company.

When following up on accounts receivables, this author writes on the patient's bill report. It is a neat and summarized way of tracking each patient's case on each report generated. So, the billing binder not only has reports printed out by case type, it has notes indicating how a balance was followed up on. Keeping these in the binder also allows one to know the last time the reports were printed and worked. The bulk of the notes about any follow-up information, however, should go into the patient's notes section of their account in the practice management software (PMS). For example:

> 4/18/08: Called United today regarding bill #22. Received notification that it wasn't received within the time frame for submission and so was denied. I have copy

> of electronic submission showing it was sent on 1/17/08 and so it should have been paid. Spoke to United today and they said they will send it back for re-processing. Ref#1222-34590999-2008. TA [initials of who made the note]

Remember that notes should follow in chronological order, the only exception to this rule is the insurance verification information that should *always* preclude any account notes at the *top* of the notes section in a patient's account for easy and frequent reference.

Annual tasks

There are many redundant end-of-the year chores that must be done with regards to insurance. *Every patient's insurance must be re-verified* at the beginning of each calendar year (there are a few policies that go July-July, those should be tagged for re-verification on August 1). Many patients' policies will change from year to year; deductibles will go up and down, patient responsibilities and co-pays can change and often the entire insurance company may have also changed. In addition, *update forms* from patients should be filled out to verify the patient's address is current and the information about their current condition is up-to-date. Getting a new copy of the patient's insurance card at the beginning of the year is important. A useful tip is to color code these forms (both the patient update and the verification form) as a quick reference to know it has been completed upon glancing at the file. For example, 2008 may be copied on yellow paper while 2009 will be on blue.

The new verification information should be noted in your PMS as described in the insurance verification section of this book.

The front desk should be aware that benefits start over at the beginning of the year and deductibles will need to be collected once again and co-pays or co-insurance amounts may have changed. If the patient has ASH, it is easy to do the first of the year verifications on-line. Simply log on and verify the patient's benefits. Be aware that if the plan changed, you may need to look up an existing patient as a *new* patient. It is generally a good practice to just look up all patients as if they were new. You can then print out these verifications on the same color paper you are using for all other verifications for that year to be consistent.

Statistics that summarize the same data as the daily and monthly statistics should be summarized on an annual basis as well. Comparing each year allows you to document the growth of your practice in each category.

In case you are wondering, there is *no* specific end-of-year tasks that must be performed relative to insurance billing. Billing and follow-up is an ongoing task that is relative to the patient's date of service, not to the calendar year.

8 Last Words

As the authors are writing this book, many, many issues are on the horizon. The national healthcare bill has passed and may have significant impact on the acupuncture profession. While this impact may be huge, it may be miniscule, and there is no way to know until it is finalized and quite possibly not for years after implementation. There is a bill in the House of Representatives to include acupuncture in Medicare and the Federal Employees Health Benefit Program (FEHBP). While the possibility of this passing may be small, if it does pass, it will have a huge impact on every single acupuncturist's practice in America. The authors of this book are keeping current with these changing policies. If any changes affect anything we have previously stated, we will make updates on our website, www.acu-insurance.com, instructing acupuncturists how to adjust your billing procedures and insurance policies accordingly.

Appendix A:
How to Deal With Individual Companies and Circumstances

Listed below is each insurance company with information specific to that company. Some insurance companies require that you must be contracted with a managed care company, such as American Specialty Health (ASH) or OptumHealth, in order to be a provider. Problems can occur between signing up for the managed care company and their informing the insurance company of your status, so one must be proactive and follow up to make sure this has happened. The system works like this: ASH or OptumHealth contract with individual insurance companies to administer their benefits. They notify the insurance companies that you are now a provider with them and for them to update their system with your information to be a provider. Information often does not get to the insurance company or the insurance company does not actually update their systems with the information given. In either case, a provider must verify their participation with each insurance company. One easy way to do this is to search for yourself in the provider database on each insurance website. If you are listed, they show you as a participating provider. If not, and you should be listed, follow up until your name shows up.

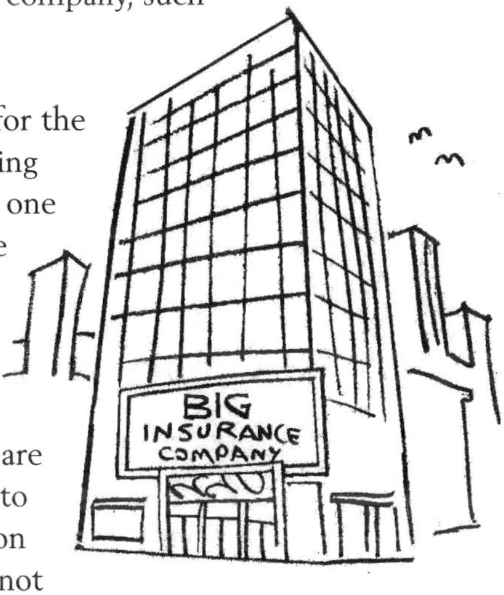

Insurance companies covered in this section of the book are listed below. These represent some of the largest insurance companies and plans that acupuncturists will be dealing with. For more information and other insurance companies, check out *www.acu-insurance.com*.

a. Aetna
b. American Specialty Health
c. Anthem (Formerly Blue Cross)
d. Blue Shield
e. Cigna
f. Health Net
g. Kaiser Permanente
h. Medi-Cal
i. Medicare
j. OptumHealth (formorly ACN)
k. Pacificare
l. Personal Injury
m. Tricare – TriWest
n. United Healthcare
o. Veterans Administration
p. Workers Compensation

Aetna

Most patients with Aetna have acupuncture coverage. In order to become an Aetna provider, you must first be an American Specialty Health (ASH) provider. Typically, an Aetna health maintenance organization (HMO) would be handled directly by ASH. A patient's insurance card would typically say HMO on it, this signals you to immediately look on www.ashlink.com (ASH's provider website) for eligibility and benefit information. A card that says PPO (preferred provider organization), would be handled directly by Aetna. A point of service (POS) plan could go either way (PPO or HMO) but more than likely, the HMO route. This should verified during the insurance verification call.

Also of extreme importance during the verification is to have them search for acupuncture benefits based specifically on the patient's group number and to determine if benefits are diagnosis specific. Aetna has gotten very specific with what diagnoses are covered and often mis-quotes benefits, quoting acupuncture coverage when they are actually dependent on the diagnosis. *You must be armed with diagnosis codes for which the patient is being treated when you call to verify coverage to see if any of them are covered.* There is also a list of these covered conditions you can print out from Aetna's website and/or they can fax it to you if you request it. It is called the "clinical policy bulletin." For example, headaches may not be covered while migraines are. Neck pain may not be covered while low back pain is. It's very specific, so to see if your patient's condition qualifies, it is recommended that you get the list.

Of Note

Aetna has some restrictions on acupuncture coverage. Always use the patient's GROUP # for benefits verification since that is where coverage may vary drastically. For many group policies, acupuncture is only covered in lieu of anesthesia or for nausea resulting from chemotherapy. Always ask the Aetna customer service rep to double check coverage and for any condition restrictions; they rarely catch the clause if you don't ask. Also, be aware of their short time frames for submission of claims (sometimes only 90 days), so follow-up must be done in a timely manner or else you risk not getting paid.

If the patient does not have acupuncture benefits but instead has a "discount plan," you must charge specific amounts or discount your charges as described by ASH. Aetna may or may not cover therapies so, as always, bill all that were done. There are no specific billing submission requirements for Aetna. This too should be asked during the verification to be sure. To summarize:

- You must be an American Specialty Health (ASH) provider to be a provider for Aetna.
- Aetna HMOs would be handled by ASH. Search for HMO eligibility on ashlink (ASH's provider website).
- Aetna PPOs are handled directly by Aetna. Call for benefit information but check ashlink first since it is easier than a phone call.
- Aetna POS would most likely be handled by ASH. Call Aetna for benefit information.
- Always ask for benefits based specifically on the patient's group number to see if benefits are dependent upon the patient's diagnosis.

American Specialty Health (ASH) –Multiple states

You must be an ASH provider to accept ASH patients. There are no out of network benefits available through ASH. By becoming an ASH provider, you become a provider for Aetna, Cigna, Anthem (Blue Cross), Kaiser, and Health Net, among others. ASH has a provider-friendly website that allows a practitioner to perform all administrative functions easily. You can verify eligibility and benefits, submit claims and clinical treatment forms for authorization, and download required forms and outcomes assessment tools among other things. When approved as a provider, you will be sent a letter along with your log-in information to access the site. You will use the website often for all activities related to ASH. Recently, ASH has begun charging a $3 fee every time they generate a paper payment (check). This fee is not charged if you are set up for direct deposit. If someone has straight ASH benefits, they typically never have a deductible, just a copay.

New providers start off with a five-visit threshold which means that you can see a patient for the first five visits without needing authorization. The exception to this is minors, age 12 and under, who need authorization from their first visit. As you become an established practitioner with ASH, they will periodically review your ability to move up in tiers which means that your treatment threshold could be increased. The next tier after five is eight; you could therefore treat a patient for the first eight visits without needing authorization and so on. For more on these tiers, contact ASH provider relations or search on ashlink. For purposes of our discussions, we will assume you are at the typical five. If a patient has been to another acupuncturist prior to seeing you and have used some of their visits, you are STILL entitled to your threshold. You do not need authorization until they have seen you for your threshold limit. You do need to be aware, however, that they have used some of their visits and should calculate how many they have remaining.

NOTE: Patients with Kaiser, using ASH to administer benefits, are not subject to this threshold. All visits must be authorized. See the Kaiser section for more information on this.

On this note, ASH has recently deemed California a "pay as you authorize" state. This means that, if they authorize visits, they are essentially counting them as used and remove them from the patient's available benefits remaining for the year. As a result, visits under authorizations not fully used by a patient, show as used visits by ASH. For example, you see a patient all year long and they have 20 visits per calendar year. You know that they have used 17 visits for the year, however, when you got authorizations throughout the year, you asked for more visits than were used. In essence, you asked for a total of 20 visits to be authorized, and they were, but the patient only used 17. Knowing this, you ask for three visits on your last authorization-so the patient can use their last three visits. ASH will deny this request stating that the patient has maxed their visits for the year. This actually isn't the case, but since they authorized all 20 already, they would need to know from which clinical treatment forms (CTFs) visits remain and you must "release" the unused visits in order to make those three available to ASH again, at which time they would reconsider your authorization request. This is done via e-mail as a reply to the denied CTF. This can be very cumbersome to the provider or the biller, to go back through each authorization and determine how many visits were authorized versus actually used to be able to ask ASH to release those unused visits. This gets even more difficult when the patient saw another provider who got authorization for more visits than used, then you have to ask the patient to call them and ask them to review their records and "release" the unused visits.

Patient visits are per calendar year. Visit thresholds, however, are July to June. This is a very complicated concept to grasp. You should track a patient's total visits by calendar year but know that their threshold starts over in July. For example, if a new patient comes to see you in February, you have a five visit threshold and therefore don't need any authorization for the first five visits. If the patient continues to come in, you will get authorizations as needed. On July 1st, if they are still treating, you now have a new threshold window of five visits where you do not need authorization. If you had gotten an authorization just prior to July, for example you requested four visits from 6/1-7/31, this is okay, but your threshold will begin *after* 7/31 since you had an authorization that spanned the new threshold time period.

When you run out of authorized visits and need to request more, you should conduct a re-examination for which you also request authorization along with the visits. You are allowed to bill a re-exam with each authorization request (if done), and to bill an initial exam with the first acupuncture treatment. You cannot conduct more than one re-exam within a 30-day time period and expect to be paid for it. If you accidentally request authorization during a threshold time period, you forfeit your right to the threshold. Always be mindful of the threshold time periods since it is your only reprieve from the authorization requirements.

You are able to charge patients for non-covered services. ASH is very specific with what your per diem rate includes: heat, E-stim, and infrared. For services that aren't included such as moxibustion, massage therapy, herbal consultations, etc. you can charge an additional fee as long as you notify the patient in advance of your intent to charge them for those services. This notification is formally acknowledged by the patient via a 'member billing acknowledgement' form (required by ASH to charge patient's additional amounts).

Sometimes a patient will have the "Acupuncture Affinity Program" through their insurance, which is only a discount program. Insurance companies who are contracted with ASH, but offer no payment for acupuncture services, receive for their members discounted rates through their affiliation. So, ASH dictates the fee limitations for acupuncture and related services through this program and one should reference ASH's website, ashlink.com, for specific fee schedules. Eligible patients will self-pay for their services. Insurance companies who participate in this program include, but are not limited to, Aetna,

Of Note

ASH has one of the most user-friendly websites of all insurance companies. Ashlink should be used for all transmissions. You can verify eligibility easily, enter claims quickly (or download a group of claims), track payments and enter clinical treatment forms. Ashlink pays you incentives for using their website, which is good, but also requires it or they will charge you an administrative fee if they have to process your paperwork manually which they will deduct from claims payments.

* New ASH providers need to sign up for the online webinar/tutorial that walks you through their site.

Health Net, and Kaiser. See ashlink for the entire list of companies who participate in this discount program. To summarize:

- You must be an ASH provider to accept ASH patients. There are *no* out of network benefits.
- ASH providers are automatically contracted with Aetna, Cigna, Blue Cross, Kaiser and HealthNet, but you should verify this with each payer.
- Use ashlink.com for all administrative tasks.
- If someone has straight ASH benefits, they typically never have a deductible, just a copay.
- New providers have a five visit threshold: you can see a patient for the first five visits without needing authorization. The threshold starts over on July 1st of each year, not January 1st.
- Benefits are by calendar year and restart at the beginning of each new year.
- New authorization requests should include a re-exam. You cannot conduct more than one re-exam within a 30 day time period and expect to be paid for it.
- All children 12 years old and younger need authorization from the first visit; they are not part of the treatment threshold policy.
- If you accidentally request authorization during a threshold time period, you forfeit your right to the threshold.
- Non-covered services can be charged as long as patients are advised in advance using ASH's "member billing acknowledgement" form.
- The "Acupuncture Affinity Program" is a discount program whereby patients are given pre-determined, discounted rates for your services. See www.ashlink.com for participants in this program and for rates.
- Denied authorizations (CTFs) citing the patient has used the maximum visits for the year, when this is not the case, need to be handled by "releasing" unused visits from prior authorizations.
- Go to *www.acu-insurance.com* for more information on forms and billing.

Anthem (formerly Blue Cross) – California and possibly other states

To be an Anthem provider, you must be contracted with American Specialty Health (ASH). Once you become contracted with ASH, you will automatically gain Anthem providership.

Most Anthem plans only cover the needling codes, no exams or therapies. You should, however, continue to bill these services since the profession is continually working on trying to add more services to our fee schedule with them. With the recent addition of two needling codes (the initial needling code 97810 or 97813 and the subsequent re-insertion codes of 97811 or 97814), you must bill Anthem *both* codes in order to get the maximum payment of $25-$33/visit (in California). So, reinsertion is necessary to get the maximum reimbursement. See the definition of reinsertion according to the current procedural terminology (CPT) codes on page 98 to determine if you are able to charge them.

If you are performing noncovered services, i.e., services not included in the primary acupuncture codes billed, (per ASH's definition since they handle the contracting), just like ASH, you may charge the patient for these non-covered services. Using the same form used for ASH patients, you must notify them in advance that you charge additional amounts for non-covered services. They should be notified and acknowledge these rates prior to treatment. There are no special billing requirements with Anthem. To summarize:

Of Note

Anthem almost always covers acupuncture and is the easiest to bill and get paid for. Unfortunately, they pay very little (~$30/visit), but at least in contrast to this, they pay for almost all conditions and do so in a reasonable timeframe. You can often verify a portion of acupuncture coverage on their website but almost always still need to call and double check the patient's benefits anyway. Anthem has a much more generous time frame for submission of claims than other payors.

- You must first be contracted with American Specialty Health (ASH) in order to be an Anthem provider.
- Most Anthem plans only cover the needling codes, not any exams or therapies.
- You may charge the patient for any noncovered services, using the same form used for ASH patients, you must notify them in advance that you charge additional amounts for noncovered services.

Blue Shield – California and possibly other states

Blue Shield is one of the few insurance companies who still handles their own contracting. You can contact Blue Shield provider relations to inquire about becoming a participating provider. The good thing about Blue Shield is that they offer more in and out of network benefits than a lot of other insurance carriers. This means that you can see a Blue Shield patient and not be a contracted provider if they have out-of-network benefits. This is not ideal, but it is an option. What this means to the provider is the patient may have a higher deductible or higher percentage responsibility for your claims as opposed to going to a contracted provider and having better benefits and less out-of-pocket responsibility. If you are an out-of-network provider, you need to be aware of the following: checks issued for services will be issued to the patient, not to the provider. Knowing this in advance you can 1) prep the patient, let them know that they will be receiving payment for your services and must bring the check to you or 2) have the patient pay your cash rates and keep the insurance check knowing that they will be reimbursed for whatever portion is covered. This is probably a better way to handle this situation unless the patient cannot afford the full fee at the time of service. Blue Shield tends to have many different policies and so reimbursements can fluctuate greatly from one patient to the next. It's almost impossible to know what they will pay until the Explanation of Benefits (EOB) is received.

Blue Shield, in approximately 70% of cases, covers some therapies and exams billed in conjunction with the primary acupuncture codes.

You should charge for all services performed and then determine what is typically allowed for that patient to know what is covered or not. To summarize:

- Blue Shield handles their own contracting; you contact them directly to become a provider and do not need to be contracted with anyone else to be a Blue Shield provider.
- Usually offers both in- and out-of-network benefits.
- If you are not an in-network provider, checks will be issued directly to the patient. You may want to have the patient pay your fees at the time of service and simply keep the insurance check instead of trying to track down the patient to get that insurance check.

Cigna

You must be contracted with ASH to be a Cigna provider. There are no specific billing requirements with Cigna. They often will pay most therapies and so you should make sure to bill all services performed.

If a patient has an HMO, any benefits would be handled directly through ASH. Cigna PPO billing goes directly to Cigna for reimbursement. To summarize:

- To be contracted with Cigna, you must first be contracted with ASH.
- HMO patients would be covered through ASH, if they have coverage.

Of Note

Cigna pays reasonably for acupuncture services and sometimes covers therapies too. If you are a participating provider with them (per your ASH contract), make sure they have you listed as such. They tend to need to be told by ASH multiple times to update their database to show you as an in-network provider. Since being in-network directly effects how the patient's benefits are applied, it's important to be listed if you are participating.

- PPO patient's bills are submitted directly to Cigna and all therapies performed should be billed since they typically pay them.

Health Net

You must be contracted with ASH to be a Health Net provider and you must treat Health Net patients just like ASH, get the same paperwork at the same intervals, request authorization when required, etc. Whether the patient has an HMO or a PPO, ASH is much more involved than with other companies. If a patient has an HMO, they would usually have benefits through ASH only, if any. You would automatically look on ashlink if a patient presented a Health Net HMO card to try and verify eligibility. If a patient has a PPO, you would still need to verify their eligibility with ASH, and if nothing comes up, call Health Net directly.

When billing, you should enter all acupuncture codes and therapies done with each treatment. Even though ASH doesn't cover therapies when billed as straight ASH, when it is a Health Net PPO the fee schedule allowance will be made for those therapies and Health Net may pay them.

ASH handles the pricing for Health Net and so ASH processes the charges, applies the allowed amounts per the applicable fee schedule and sends this "pricing sheet" to Health Net who then issues the recommended payment. This is why you should enter all therapies done, because Health Net should pay for them if they are on their fee schedule. For services that aren't included such as moxibustion, massage therapy, herbal consultations, etc. you can charge additional fees utilizing the same system and paperwork as for ASH; the member billing acknowledgement form.

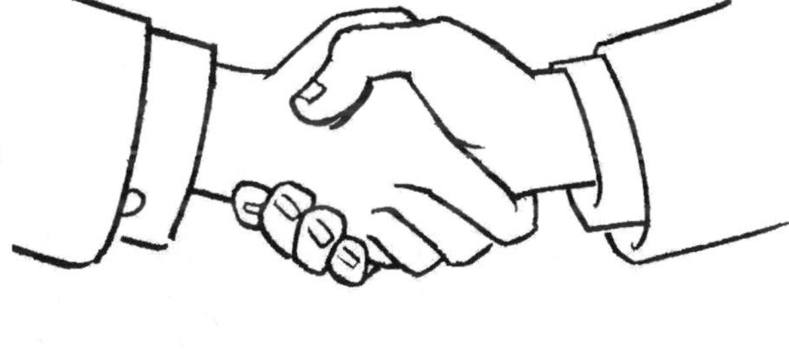

To summarize:

- ASH providers are automatically contracted with Health Net
- You must use the same paperwork, authorization process if required, etc., for Health Net as you do for ASH.
- All Health Net claim submissions must be done via ashlink whether it is an HMO or PPO plan.
- All charges should be entered for this payer as they may pay for more than just the acupuncture codes.

Kaiser Permanente

To be a Kaiser provider, you must be contracted with ASH. Kaiser is an HMO, so there would never be any other type of benefits (such as PPO) available. Many Kaiser plans provide acupuncture coverage, however, a referral must be obtained prior to treatment and must come, not from the primary treating physician, but specifically from the pain management clinic.

The process works like this. The patient goes to the pain management clinic at Kaiser, where the doctor determines acupuncture would be an appropriate treatment and writes a referral for acupuncture. This referral gets sent to ASH. ASH then sends the patient a letter, stating that they've received a referral and the patient must do three things:

1. Find an acupuncture provider. It may say that a provider has been selected for you. If one has been selected, it lists the name, address and phone number of the acupuncturist. If not, the patient goes to www.ashcompanies.com and chooses one or calls ASH to help them select one. If the patient wants to change acupuncturists, they simply inform ASH of the change; they do NOT need to go back to Kaiser.
2. Call to schedule an appointment. The patient should take this referral letter with them to their appointment and the provider should make a copy of it to keep in the patient's file.
3. Receive treatment. The referral begins with a trial of five treatments. After the five, an assessment of the patient's progress

should be performed and more treatments may be requested by completing a CTF (Clinical Treatment Form), thereby requesting authorization from ASH.

The Kaiser referral is good for one year. The authorization process (through ASH) continues for the next year until the referral expires. After one year, the patient must return to the pain management clinic at Kaiser for a new referral, if required. Just remember that the acupuncturist must only reference the condition on the referral when seeking authorization from ASH. To summarize:

- Kaiser is handled directly through ASH. See review of ASH procedures under the ASH heading of this book.
- You must have a referral from the pain management clinic at Kaiser in order to see the patient. A referral is good for one year.
- You can search for a patient's referral on ashlink.com and should print it out for your records.
- After verifying the referral, the patient has five visits before needing to request authorization from ASH again.
- Billing is done via ashlink.com as is typical with ASH.
- Use ashlink.com for all administrative tasks.

Medi-Cal

Medi-Cal is a California state funded insurance program for low-income people. It stopped paying for acupuncture in March of 2009 due to the economy. The following information is included in case the program is reinstated in the future. Please keep an eye on the authors' website for updates.

Visits were limited to two per calendar month and you had to be a contracted provider to see Medi-Cal patients. Treatment was limited to the prevention or alleviation of severe, persistent, chronic pain resulting from a generally recognized medical condition. Eligibility had to be re-verified monthly though no prescription was required. The fee schedule is listed below and the reimbursements were very low. The billing and follow-up efforts were very high. Although an MD referral to treat was not required for Medi-Cal the authors suggest you analyze the cost effectiveness of becoming a provider before doing so should this be offered again in the future. When billing, there was a six month time limit for filing and collecting on claims. To ensure accurate reimbursement for all acupuncture services, claims needed to include the diagnosis of the condition causing the pain, other treatments given, and results of other treatments. Billable CPT codes are listed below. After the creation of a second acupuncture code to be billed with the primary code (the first insertion of needles [97810] and the re-insertion [97811]), providers were paid a maximum reimbursement of $11.58 per visit if both codes were performed and billed. However, due to the current situation of Medi-Cal and acupuncture, we will not cover how to bill it here. For information on billing Medi-Cal, should it be covered in the future, please visit our website: *www.acu-insurance.com.*

To summarize:

- Providers must be contracted with Medi-Cal to treat Medi-Cal patients
- Patients were limited to 2 visits per calendar month when the plan covered acupuncture

Medi-Cal Codes and Rates

CPT-4 Code	Description	Maximum Allowance
97810	Acupuncture, one or more needles, without electrical stimulation; initial 15 minutes	$5.79
97811	Acupuncture, one or more needles, without electrical stimulation; each additional 15 minutes **of personal one-on-one contact with the patient, with reinsertion of needle(s)**	$5.79
97813	Acupuncture, one or more needles, with electrical stimulation; initial 15 minutes **of personal one-on-one contact with the patient**	$5.79
97814	Acupuncture, one or more needles, with electrical stimulation; each additional 15 minutes **of personal one-on-one contact with the patient, with reinsertion of needle(s)**	$5.79

- Acupuncturists are limited to treatment of pain relating to generally recognized medical conditions.
- Must re-verify eligibility monthly.
- No prescription is required to treat
- There is a 6 month billing time limit for all claims
- Make sure to include the diagnosis of the condition causing the pain, other treatments given
- Medi-Cal does not cover acupuncture at the time of publication of this book.

Medicare

A federally funded medical insurance program to cover those 65 years of age and older, Medicare does not offer coverage for acupuncture currently. At the time this is written, bills have been proposed to Congress that would include the payment of acupuncture but are unlikely to pass as they have not in previous attempts. However, some insurers (in lieu of Medicare) offer acupuncture benefits but operate as HMOs and therefore you must be contracted in order to utilize any benefits.

Just because Medicare doesn't cover acupuncture at the present time does not mean that you will never have to deal with them, unfortunately. First of all, when doing an insurance verification on a patient 65 years of age or older, you must be very careful to make sure they do not have Medicare. Most patients have other insurance in addition to Medicare or instead of Medicare. When insurance is in addition to Medicare, it can cover: 1) Medicare's deductibles and copays, but *must* be a benefit payable by Medicare before it will provide any coverage, this is referred to as a "supplemental" policy (and would *not* cover acupuncture) or 2) the insurance could be a completely separate, full coverage secondary insurance. In this case, you could potentially use this insurance if there was acupuncture coverage.

The other possibility is that the patient "opted out" of straight Medicare and gave up their benefits for another policy which is usually an HMO. Rarely is there acupuncture coverage through this type of policy, although it is becoming slightly more common. The benefit for patients to do this is usually because the HMO offers more prescription drug coverage than regular Medicare does, which can be important for older patients. You will have to deal with Medicare when there is a completely separate, full coverage policy that covers acupuncture.

To bill a secondary insurance that has acupuncture coverage, you will have to show that the primary payor (Medicare) does NOT cover acupuncture. To do this, there is an easy way and a hard way. Obviously you want to do it the easy way and should try it first. Unfortunately, sometimes the insurance won't recognize this and will insist you do it the hard way.

1. The *easy way*: Send, with your bills to the secondary insurance, a copy from Medicare's provider manual the statement that acupuncture is not a covered benefit under Medicare. See our website for a copy of this page that you can print out and send with your claims.
2. The *hard way*: After you've tried to send what should be an obvious explanation about Medicare's policy of not covering acupuncture, the secondary may still insist on seeing a denial from the primary payor (Medicare). You will need to actually get a denial from Medicare. To get a denial from Medicare you will need to send your bills to Medicare first. Unfortunately, since you are not in their system (and cannot be since acupuncturists are not contracted with them), they will *not* automatically kick back a denial to you. You must wait about two weeks to 30 days after submitting your claim to *call* Medicare and ask them to *manually deny* your claim. This will prompt them to send you a denial, at which time you can copy it and send it in with your claim to the secondary insurance company. This is a cumbersome process and is not one you would deal with often, if that is any consolation.
   To summarize:

- Acupuncture is *not* covered by Medicare at this time.
- If the patient has a secondary insurance, carefully verify it to make sure it covers acupuncture and is not just a supplemental to Medicare.
- You will need to submit either the explanation from Medicare that acupuncture is not covered or get a denial from Medicare to copy and send to the secondary along with your claim(s).

- Verifying coverage can be very difficult to figure out since Medicare requires adults to have Medicare once they reach age 65. Many different insurance options are then made available in addition to or in lieu of Medicare so make sure to verify all coverage involved.

OptumHealth (Formerly ACN)

OptumHealth not only handles contracting for Pacificare, United Healthcare, and Great West, they now, in many instances, pay claims on their behalf as well. When verifying benefits for these payors, you should verify where to send claims. OptumHealth has a set fee schedule for the initial acupuncture visit versus follow-up visits. Fee schedules should be mailed to you when you become a provider and you should also be able to access them at their provider website.
To summarize:

- OptumHealth is formerly ACN, although both names are still used.
- OptumHealth handles Pacificare, United Healthcare and Great West contracting as well as some claim processing.

Pacificare (currently changing to United Healthcare)

To be contracted with Pacificare, you must be contracted with OptumHealth. Depending on the information obtained during insurance verification, the patient may or may not have in/out of network benefits which will determine if you are able to see the patient based on your provider status with Pacificare. If the patient's policy is a PPO then billing will be done directly through Pacificare. However, if the patient's policy is an HMO, then billing will go through OptumHealth. Pacificare and United Healthcare merged and are part of the same company so you may see both names on correspondence. Now Pacificare is changing its name entirely to United Healthcare and soon that is the only name you will see. There are no special billing requirements for this payor regardless of PPO or HMO status. You should bill all therapies done with the treatment since they sometimes pay therapies in addition to the needling codes. If it's an HMO, this is not typically the case; usually they pay one flat per-diem rate, much like ASH. To summarize:

- There are no special billing requirements for this payer.
- Bill all therapies done in conjunction with the acupuncture codes for possible payment.
- PPO plans are billed directly to Pacificare, HMO plans are billed to OptumHealth.
- Pacificare and United Healthcare are related.

Personal injury (PI)

Personal injury cases are either auto accidents or less often, slip and fall type accidents. These cases can be paid by health insurance, med-pay, and/or attorneys or any combination thereof. PI cases are not for everyone; they require meticulous record keeping, an element of risk, and extra aggravation from dealing with opposing lawyers and the court system. However, they can be monetarily rewarding, with large payoffs at your highest treatment rates. Because they are so risky and yet potentially lucrative, the authors urge practitioners to attempt them, but create limits. Don't take too many of these cases as they can take a lot of time and may not be fully resolved, or paid, for years. But a few in a case load create some diversity and potential rewards.

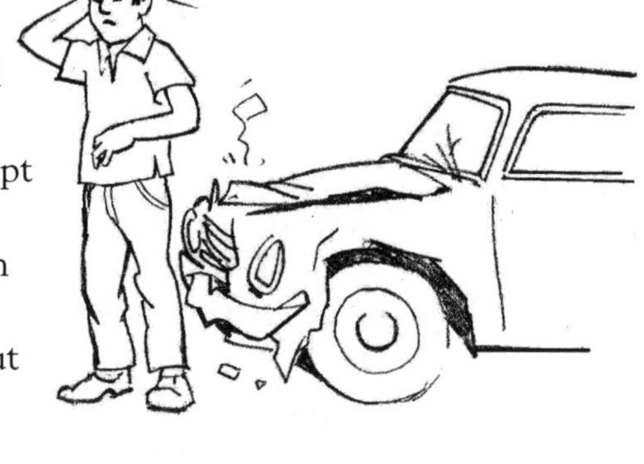

Personal injury cases are specific to an accident and record keeping needs to be very accurate including proper outcome assessments. Paperwork needs to be in order as you will typically be called upon to write reports regarding the patient's condition and may even be called upon to testify in court. The records will be copied multiple times so the legal system can determine who owes what to whom. The documentation must be in tip top shape. In California, there is a two year statute of limitations to settle or file a suit (from the date of accident). Keep this in mind as the patient is treated. If nothing has progressed on the case after two years, the responsible party is no longer held liable for the accident. If you are not in California, make sure to familiarize yourself with your state's statutory timeframes.

There are various levels of risk associated with PI cases; determining this at the onset is integral to your decision to take a particular case. You should exercise due diligence to find out details of the accident. Request the accident report from the patient right away. This usually documents who was determined to be at fault. If your patient was found to be at fault, unless they have health insurance or med-pay, the other party will not take responsibility and so no attorney will take the case. Once you are able to determine that the patient was *not* at fault, you then need to know how much damage was done to their car. If damage is minimal, less than $1,000, it is not a good case. If damage is less than $1,500 the case is shaky but if the damage is above $1,500 the case should be good.

There are still other considerations prior to determining the viability of a case. The type of damage is important, if it's just a bumper, then even if it costs $2,500 to repair, the case still won't be looking to handle very much in medical bills. If damage is to the frame or other parts of the car besides the bumper, and the repair costs are greater than $1,500, the case should be able to sustain a decent amount of medical bills, assuming they are medically necessary and documented accordingly.

You want to also make sure you are treating the patient within a reasonable timeframe of the accident. As a general rule, if the patient's accident was more than three months prior to when they first seek treatment, this raises red flags. You will need to justify why, if the patient was so badly injured, they were able to go without treatment for so long without needing care. Although this can be easily explained (for example, the patient tried to use over the counter pain medications hoping it would resolve but it didn't, or the symptoms slowly progressed to an unmanageable level, etc.), you will need to be able to justify the need for treatment. This can be a concern and you should be prepared to explain it. If the patient has an attorney, it is a good idea to talk to the attorney at the onset of treatment and ask about the case to determine how much they recommend for medical billing; basically, how much medical cost the case can handle. They are also privy to how much medical care the patient may have already received, *i.e.* hospital bills, ambulance bills, etc. which may impact how much you should treat the patient (and expect to get paid). Part of your due diligence is making sure you get the third party information even if the patient has med-pay, health insurance, or an attorney. Things can go bad with cases (more on this below) and having *all* information arms you with the best chance of collecting on your bill. There are also different PI payment types:

Med-pay/Personal Injury Protection (PIP). Med-pay (or PIP; personal injury protection as it is sometimes called) is a benefit that people can have on their own auto insurance policies that pay medical bills if they are involved in an auto accident. In the authors' opinion, everyone should have med-pay since it is an inexpensive way to ensure medical coverage if one is involved in an accident and needs medical care. Providers are able to bill the med-pay and get paid for their medical bills right away. When a patient is involved in an auto accident, you want to verify that they have med-pay coverage and know that it is the preferred method of payment for PI cases. Although med-pay typically covers all services, rarely they will exclude acupuncture. Call and verify that acupuncture is a covered service under the patient's med-pay.

Med-pay usually covers a driver and their passengers, usually to a maximum of six passengers–verification of the policy provisions would be necessary for limitations.

If a patient says they were a passenger in an auto accident, you will want to try and verify if the driver had med-pay first and, if not, if the patient themselves had med-pay coverage through their own auto insurance policy.

Med-pay excess means that med-pay covers the excess after a patient's health insurance has been billed. Prior to billing the med pay, you must bill the patient's health insurance. Once you receive the explanation of benefits (EOB) back, then the bill must be sent to the med-pay with a *copy* of that EOB. Most med-pay policies cover the patient's responsibility portion so if the visit was mostly paid by the health insurance and a copay, coinsurance, or deductible was withheld, the med pay will only pay those patient responsibility amounts. Some companies may pay the balance that was billed but not paid. If the patient does not have health insurance, but has med pay excess, you will need to have them sign a statement that they do not have health insurance at this time. This is a simple letter but if you would like to see an example, go to our website.

Patient confusion about their med pay benefits and being obstinate about using it is sometimes a hurdle. First, make sure you have an explanation about med pay in your PI Payment Policy form that patient's should be signing which acknowledges their understanding of your policies. For a sample form that is customizable, please see our website. There is a fear that when a patient uses their med pay benefits, their premiums will increase, especially if the accident was not their fault and the other party is taking responsibility for payment of their bills. This is not true:

1. Med-pay is a benefit that you *pay* for and should therefore be *used* when the time is appropriate.
2. Premiums *do not* increase when it is used (in California, it is against the law to raise your rates if you were not at fault). If you were at fault, your premiums may go up because you are accessing your insurance.
3. Upon settlement of your claim, the responsible person's insurance will have to negotiate with the med pay at the conclusion of the case to *reimburse* them for monies spent for the patient's medical care it paid out when it, technically, was not their responsibility to pay.
4. As a patient, you want to be able to get the medical care you need, when you need it, following an accident and not all providers accept liens (more on this next).

Basically, med-pay is a fund that fronts the medical bills until it gets reimbursed at the end of the case by the responsible party. If the patient was at fault, they can still use their med-pay. As a provider, you prefer med-pay because you get paid right away for your services and do not have to wait until the case settles which can take up to two years. If there is no attorney on the case, you risk not getting paid at all.

If you have an issue with an attorney trying to control a patient's med-pay, go to our website for troubleshooting and recommendations on how to handle this infrequent issue.

PI Liens. Also, known as Attorney Liens, this is a legally binding document that a patient and their attorney signs acknowledging the need to pay your bill out of the pending PI settlement. When a patient comes in for a PI case, they should sign a lien (for a lien you can customize, go to our website). This lien should be signed by the patient even if they don't have an attorney yet and kept in their file. If and when they do have an attorney, this lien should be faxed to their attorney for signature. If they don't have a fax machine, keep a *copy* of this lien and mail them the original. Keep notes to follow-up until it is received back; only when it is signed and returned is it valid. Keep this in the patient's file. Sometimes attorneys will amend the lien, cross out a line here or there or handwrite something in. You will need to assess the changes that were made, see how significantly (or not) it affects the lien, and decide if it's something you can live with. If you still disagree with the changes, you are not obligated to accept them, call the attorney and try to work it out.

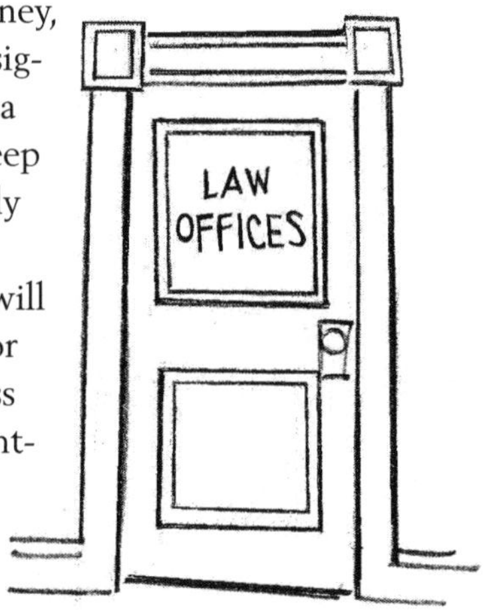

At the conclusion of the treatment, the final bill should be sent to the attorney along with a short letter stating that the patient has concluded treatment with you and ask if they would like chart notes and/or a report. Reports are typically charged and added to the bill (with the report you would send an amended bill). If the PI case seems to be taking some time to settle, you will want to contact the attorney's office periodically to check on the status of the case. Note that in California, the statute of limitations to either settle a claim or file a lawsuit is two years and sometimes these PI cases can take up until that two year mark to settle or, at that point, file a lawsuit. Usually attorneys take that time to try and resolve the case prior to filing suit. Typically, payment on a PI case can take at least six months following the conclusion of treatment. You should keep on top of these cases and not assume that your bill will be handled sometime in the distant future because things can go wrong. For instance, the patient could fire their attorney or, more likely, the attorney could drop the patient as a client. Either of these scenarios does not happen very often, however, when it does, you are back to a third-party lien situation which is a bad place to be, more on this in the next section.

When it is finally time to settle the PI case, don't be surprised if you get a call from the attorney's office requesting you to take a bill reduction, it is a common practice. As the practitioner, you have the option of reducing your bill or not. The authors typically ask for a reason to reduce the bill; you should not have to arbitrarily reduce the bill unless the settlement was not very good in relation to the outstanding medical bills, etc. It is perfectly fine to ask how much the settlement was and request a list of disbursements. Note that you should always bill for all services you perform such as therapies, exams, etc. in conjunction with the acupuncture codes so that your full bill is considered. This also gives you a little more leeway to reduce your bill in the end, if necessary.

Third Party PI Situations/Liens. The term "lien" here is grossly misleading since they are by no means binding, like a standard PI attorney lien is. It is a huge problem for healthcare providers since a third party lien is *not* legally binding.

Basically, this is what you end up with when a PI patient has no attorney, no med-pay, and no health insurance. They have been told by the third party (insurance for the responsible party involved in the accident) that they will pay for the patient's medical bills at the conclusion of treatment. The problem is this: *who* will they pay for the medical bills? To try and protect yourself, you have the patient sign a third party lien that *directs* the third party to pay you directly for their medical bills at the conclusion of treatment. Although you have this form signed, the third party is not legally bound to honor it. Sometimes they will say if you have the patient call and ask them to cut a check directly to you, then and only then will they do so. Sometimes they still don't pay you directly. Here is the reality of the situation: their insured hit your patient in an auto accident. As the insurance company for the responsible party, their obligation is to the patient to cover damages incurred as a result of the accident; not to all of the providers from whom the patient sought care. It becomes the ultimate responsibility of the patient to pay their debts to medical providers. In the end, most of the time, in spite of all your efforts to avoid the inevitable, the insurance will send payment for your medical bill to the patient, coupled with any pain and suffering or other expenses being paid to the patient to resolve the claim with their insured. At this point, it is between you and your patient to get paid. Often times and very unfortunately, patients do not pay their bills. These can be the nicest of patients who used to come in to the office and bring you baked goods, etc. and you thought for sure you could trust to pay their bill. You would be shocked to know how many people skip on their bill. For this reason, these authors have a strict policy in the office of *not* accepting third party liens; we simply can't afford to. Of course it's always up to you to make that decision. There are some good patients out there who can be trusted but be very, very cautious with whom you allow this situation. If you are going to allow a third party lien, it is very important that they sign an acknowledgement of their responsibility to pay you from any settlement they receive.

Remember too that you can end up in a situation like this if a patient's attorney dropped their case somewhere along the way. This is another reason why it's always important to get *all* information at the beginning of a case including the third party information – this scenario actually occurs more often than you might think. In the event of a third party situation you need to be able to call the third party insurance and ask for the status of the case so you know exactly when a case settled and when the patient got their payment so that you can immediately pursue the patient for payment before they spend it. It is also within your right to ask the third party insurance company how much they allowed for your medical bill. This way you know if your bill was reduced or not and exactly what you should request from the patient for your medical bills. There is one other situation that you could encounter; in California it's called a Prop 213. This is when the

person who was hit had no auto insurance. Even though someone else is responsible for the damages to their car, because they had no auto insurance of their own, they cannot collect pain and suffering from the person who hit them. The insurance can and will only pay for their medical care. Sometimes in these cases, the insurance will agree more readily to pay the provider directly. This arrangement should be in writing with the third party insurance company but is still not an absolute guarantee of direct payment. If the payment goes to the patient in this case, without receiving any other monies for pain and suffering, it can be even more difficult to get the money from the patient since all they received is payment for their medical bills.
To summarize:

- It is highly recommended that you do not attempt to treat a PI case until reading this entire section – the summary cannot fully impart the depth of knowledge you should have to treat and get paid for a PI case.
- PI cases are often the result of auto accidents; less often slip and falls.
- An MD referral is NOT necessary for a patient to receive acupuncture for a PI case.
- Determining financial responsibility for the case is the first order of business. A patient may have health insurance, med pay, med-pay excess, or an attorney (or none of these). Payment could come from one or a combination of these. All payment methods should be verified with med pay being the preferred form of payment for all PI cases as it is the easiest and fastest way to get paid.
- If the patient has no method of payment and was not at fault, you have a third party lien situation. These are highly risky since you are essentially relying on the patient to receive payment of your bill directly and kindly forward it on to you. This often does not happen smoothly. The term "lien" is used loosely as there is no legally binding obligation for anyone to pay you, just a form called a lien that you hope everyone will honor during settlement. Payment of your bill almost always goes to the patient.
- If the patient has no method of payment and was at fault, you have a cash patient requiring diligently documented treatment notes. The only way this will be recognizable as a PI case is your

note taking. You should charge and receive your cash rates as the patient is treated since no one else will pay. This is the only time you should charge cash rates for a PI case.

- Determine the viability of the case; get the accident report, find out how much damage was done, if the third party accepted liability, etc. This information will help you decide if the case is strong (or not), how much it is reasonable to bill and, more importantly, what amount would be excessive.
- Your documentation must be thorough as it could be entered into legal proceedings or you could be called upon to testify.
- If the patient presents to you without an attorney, have them sign an Attorney lien anyway. It will be kept in their file for execution in the event they later retain an attorney. It's nearly impossible to get the patient to sign a lien after they've been released from care.
- Make sure to charge for all services performed; do not simply charge your cash rate. If you applied heat packs and did some massage in conjunction with your treatments, bill it. In the end, as is the case with most PI cases, the attorney will ask you to reduce a portion of your bill. You want to have as much leeway as possible to reduce your bill. You should also ask why a reduction is being requested, it is not automatic (although it seems that way).

TriCare – TriWest

Currently there are no benefits. Charge cash rates. You may offer a military discount if you like and it is clearly defined in your fee schedule.

United Healthcare

You must be contracted with OptumHealth in order to be contracted with United Healthcare. Bill all services performed since sometimes they consider other therapies for payment. There are no special billing requirements with this payor. There are HMO and PPO plans with this payor, which will determine where you submit your claims. This will be determined when you verify the patient's insurance and claims submission information. To summarize:

- There are no special billing requirements with this payor.
- Bill all services performed since sometimes they consider therapies.

Of Note

United Healthcare only pays for acupuncture codes and does so at a reasonable rate (they used to cover some therapies, but no longer do). Beware of their limited timeframes for submission! Sometimes their timeframes are as low as 90 days, follow-up must be timely or else you risk not getting paid.

Veterans Administration (VA)

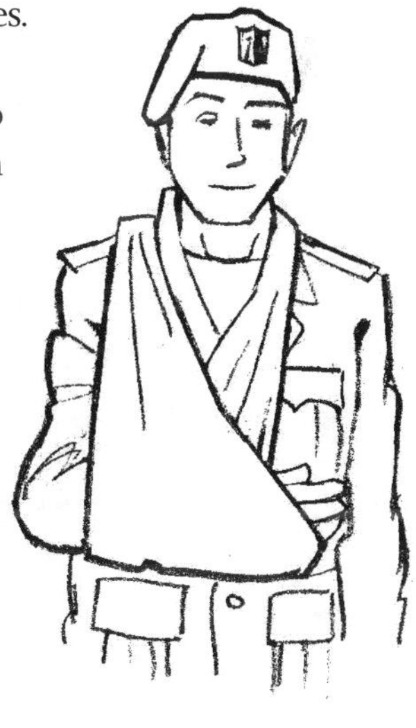

You do not need to be contracted with anyone in particular to accept VA as insurance. What you do need is prior authorization in writing. When a patient receives an authorization for acupuncture, usually the only designation is that you are an acupuncturist within the county where they received the authorization and VA services. Always review the authorization prior to initiating a course of treatment to ensure that you are allowed to treat the patient (a specific acupuncturist hasn't been designated other than you, for example), the number of treatments authorized and valid dates to provide treatment along with the diagnosis code for which they are being referred. The diagnosis on the authorization should match your claim. If, at the conclusion of treatment, you believe the patient should receive additional treatment, you can request another authorization (following the submission directions on the original authorization form). Never treat without a valid authorization. Billing information should also be listed on the original authorization and may instruct you to submit chart notes and/or other medical documentation with your bills. You should include all services performed on your bill. The first time you submit billing to the VA, they will send you paperwork to set you up as a vendor in their system. They will request such information as a W-9 and a few general forms to be completed regarding you and your practice prior to processing your bills. Subsequent to this, you will be in their system and able to submit bills with no delay in processing. To summarize:

- You do not need to be contracted with the VA to bill acupuncture.
- You do need to get prior authorization before administering treatment.
- Always scrutinize the authorization for treatment details and dates, instructions, billing addresses, etc. since the VA is very strict about not paying for any treatment not authorized, provided within their stipulated timeframes, or an unauthorized diagnosis.

Workers' Compensation

Workers' compensation (work comp for short) provides insurance coverage to employees who were injured while on the job. Most states' workers comp systems have gone through dramatic overhauls due to difficult financial times. You should look into your individual state's work comp laws for specific guidelines. You can also reference our website for work comp information by state at *www.acu-insurance.com*. Regardless of the rules, there is one constant procedure that, if you follow, should always result in a paying work comp claim. Get prior authorization, in writing. This is absolutely imperative to ensure you get your claim paid. Next, make sure you do not bill for a condition other than the one caused by the work injury and that has been authorized.

In some states, such as California, most insurance carriers require you to belong to their "MPN" or medical provider network in order to treat their patients. Generally, you cannot receive an authorization if you are not on the MPN list. Conversely, if you want to receive referrals, you will need to get on the list so you are an option when they choose an acupuncturist to refer to. More information on MPNs below.

Claims submission requirements should be asked about during the verification process. Typically, office notes and/or reports may be required with claim submissions and almost always to justify an initial exam charge that accompanies acupuncture charges on the first visit and at re-exams. Since the collection of specific information is so important for a workers' comp patient, the procedures to follow prior to the patients arrival and once they arrive has been detailed below.

Before a patient arrives: Usually if a patient is workers' comp, they will say so when they call to schedule their appointment because, typically, they would have gotten a prescription or (hopefully) an authorization to treat already and were referred to you specifically. While scheduling the patient or while making a reminder phone call, you should tell the patient to bring the following information with them to their first appointment:

- Their adjuster's information
- Prescription from their primary treating physician for acupuncture
- If obtained, the authorization information

If there isn't an authorization yet, you need to get this prior to initiating a course of treatment. Also let them know that there is quite a bit of paperwork to complete prior to their appointment so ask them to come early and be prepared with their case information. You could also mail the paperwork in advance or have forms on your website.

When the patient arrives:

- You will need the patient to complete a work comp specific questionnaire that addresses the details of the work injury. It is helpful to get, at least, the primary treating physician's latest report to help better understand the patient's condition.
- You should get a copy of the patient's driver's license to keep in their file. You should now collect their prescription for acupuncture, their work comp payer information including the adjusters name and contact information, the patient's claim number, and date of injury (DOI). This information will also be collected when you complete the work comp verification form (see below).

- A fee schedule and HIPAA form should also be signed and filed.
- The patient should complete the appropriate pain questionnaires on the first visit, prior to treatment. This establishes a baseline of the patient's condition and helps show positive treatment outcomes for further authorization.
- Once an authorization has been used, you must be able to document medical improvement—which is done via outcomes assessments—to prove that the patient has positively responded to your treatment. This supports your request for additional authorization. It can sometimes be helpful and even necessary to give the patient a copy of the previous, completed outcome assessment so they can more accurately complete the subsequent one.

Medical Provider Networks (MPNs). While not in every state, MPNs are the *umbrella* group that you must belong to, to access the insurance company beneath it. For example, you must belong to the Medrisk MPN in order to treat patients with the following insurances: Liberty Mutual, Sedgwick, etc. In the case of Medrisk, you actually bill them directly. You need to contact each MPN to determine claims submission and who handles authorizations, etc.

For more information about joining an MPN, go to our website, *www.acu-insurance.com*, where you can click on links directly to the MPN you are interested in joining. It also lists which MPN each insurance company is affiliated with. While many MPNs are full, there are still quite a few that are accepting new providers.

A Work Comp verification form is used to verify a patient's billing information and should include the claim number, date of injury, insurance company name and address for claims, the adjuster's name, phone and fax numbers along with the utilization review's phone and fax numbers. Verify that the claim is open and active as well. If there is an attorney on the case, you should get their information, too.

Authorization and payment protection recommendations. With regards to workers' compensation cases, you have some recourse if the insurance company messes with you. First, protect yourself and always get authorization before initiating a course of acupuncture treatment, in writing. In most covered states, you must get authorization from the adjuster or review company prior to rendering treatment anyway, so get it in writing. If you do not, you run the risk of not getting paid. Sometimes adjusters give verbal authorization over the phone, after which any number of things can happen. The person leaves the company and the new adjuster does not see any record of that authorization, so they won't pay your claim(s). An adjuster may forget that they ever gave authorization, didn't make any notes, and, therefore, won't pay your claim(s). A new adjuster may be assigned to the claim who goes by a different set of rules and doesn't think the patient should have acupuncture at all for their condition! They may say that they did not realize you were an acupuncture clinic when they gave the authorization and, had they known, never would have authorized the treatment at all. By the way, these are all experiences the authors have had. So, protect yourself and always get authorization in writing. If they don't have anything to send to you, write up a quick blurb stating that per your conversation they have authorized x number of visits, etc., fax it to them and request it be signed and sent back. Hold firm to this procedure so you do not get burned.

Another good reason for this practice is that, once the bills are being processed by bill review, they may not have a record of the authorization and deny the claims for lack of it. Only when you have it in writing can you resubmit the claims with a copy of the authorization as proof, which cannot be argued.

If the work comp company still refuses to pay your claims you can do a few things:

1. Have the patient call to inquire about why their provider hasn't been paid
2. Call the adjuster's supervisor explaining how you had authorization in advance of treatment and so there is no reason why your claims should not be paid.
3. Call the patient's attorney, if they have one, and see if they can apply pressure for you.
4. File a "notice and request for allowance of lien" form. See the WCAB (Workers' Comp Appeals Board) website for forms.

A work comp lien is a medical lien attached to a worker's comp claim.

Patients with a "lifetime" award. Once there were the days when a patient was awarded a final settlement on their work comp claim with the addition of lifetime medical care they could actually use for treatment. Some even took the medical care only, because they would need future treatment, in lieu of part of their financial settlement. The current problem with this is that you are not automatically entitled to the "award" you were granted. Medical necessity and prior authorization must be received, in addition to documenting what *flared* this patient's work comp injury. Sometimes, if this verbiage of "flaring" is not included, the request will be denied. The medical care allowance in a final work comp award would be written in the patient's P&S report (permanent and stationary) which is done at the conclusion of the patient's case and is the law for all future care. If a patient is coming to you for treatment of an old work comp case, you would need to know if they have the ability to even see an acupuncturist as this would have been stipulated in the future medical care section of their P&S. The patient should have a copy of their award and P&S report.

If you follow the rules of authorization specified in this section, you should be fine. This way, the adjuster determines if acupuncture is covered, based on the lifetime medical award, and can make the decision to authorize acupuncture treatment or not. If the patient believes they have acupuncture and the adjuster denies the authorization, scrutinize their P&S report, and review the future medical care section. If you find acupuncture listed, you can cite this in your rebuttal to the adjuster for acupuncture authorization. If the patient still has an attorney involved in their case, they can be very helpful in applying pressure to ensure that the patient gets their awarded medical benefits, again assuming in this case that acupuncture is specifically listed as a future medical treatment option.

Work comp authorization process. First, a patient must get a prescription (Rx) for acupuncture from their primary treating physician. That physician's office may forward their report and Rx to the insurance company and obtain authorization for the services prior to the patient ever seeking treatment from you. This is always nice and very helpful but only happens in about 50% of the cases. The other 50% are handled like this; the patient has received an Rx for acupuncture from

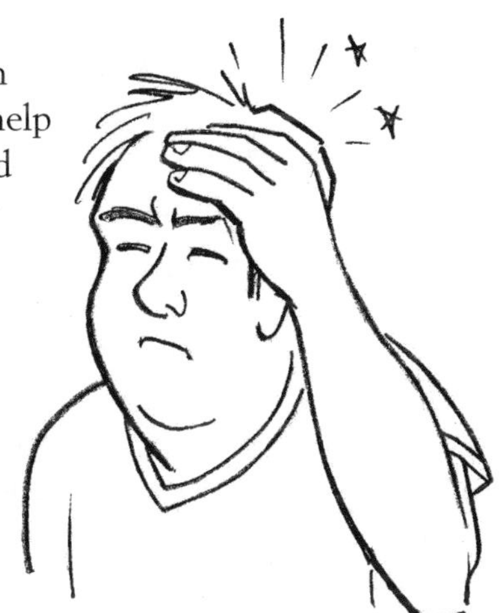

their primary physician and calls you to get an appointment. At this point, you will need to help facilitate the authorization process. You should fax the prescription to the insurance company and follow-up with the patient's adjuster.

Once you complete an authorization and want to request another, you need to write a report documenting the patient's current condition, treatment response (as evidenced by your outcome assessments), goals attained from treatment and current goals of continued treatment. You then fax this report to both the primary physician as well as the insurance adjuster or Utilization Review [UR] department. The adjuster or UR department may authorize more visits based on your report but most often will require a new Rx from the primary physician. Since you faxed your report to the primary physician's office also, if they agree with your course of treatment, they can easily write another Rx and hopefully help to get your authorization approved. Of course, this process is much easier if you have done proper outcomes assessments throughout the treatment process. To summarize:

- It is highly recommended that you do not attempt work comp until reading this entire section – the summary cannot fully impart the depth of knowledge you should have to treat and get paid for work comp patients.
- Check your state's work comp laws; they vary from state to state.
- Always get authorization in writing. If a written authorization cannot be provided, write it up yourself and fax it to the adjuster for their signature.
- Make certain that the body parts you are treating are, in fact, covered under your patient's work comp case. Do not ever diagnose and treat an unrelated body part from the approved condition as it has not been substantiated as work related unless accepted by the employer and work comp carrier.

- You must get on MPN lists! Participation in Medical Provider Networks is a must to be able to treat and maintain work comp patients in the states that require it.
- Patients should arrive early to their first appointment to complete all paperwork and to provide you with all necessary information such as insurance and adjuster information, Rx, claim number,etc.
- The use of pain questionnaires and outcomes assessments to document your treatment's success provides the necessary medical justification for subsequent authorization requests. Always have the patient complete the initial one prior to the first treatment to establish a baseline. After that, they should complete subsequent questionnaires at re-exams. Giving patients a copy of their previous form can be helpful so they recall what they answered before.
- Lifetime awards are specific for future medical care. The patient would have to have acupuncture listed as part of future medical care and still, it would have to be pre-authorized.
- Always stay in communication with the primary treating physician. Send them copies of all reports you send to the insurance company.

Medical provider networks for workers compensation

- Blue Cross
- Broadspire
- Corvel
- Coventry
- ESIS
- Hartford
- Liberty Mutual
- Pinnacol Assurance
- Sedgwick
- Specialty Risk Services (SRS)
- State Compensation Insurance Fund (SCIF)
- Travelers
- Tristar
- Zenith

Checking out Mpnfinder.com or www.acu-insurance.com are excellent resources for more MPNs.

Appendix B: Sample Forms

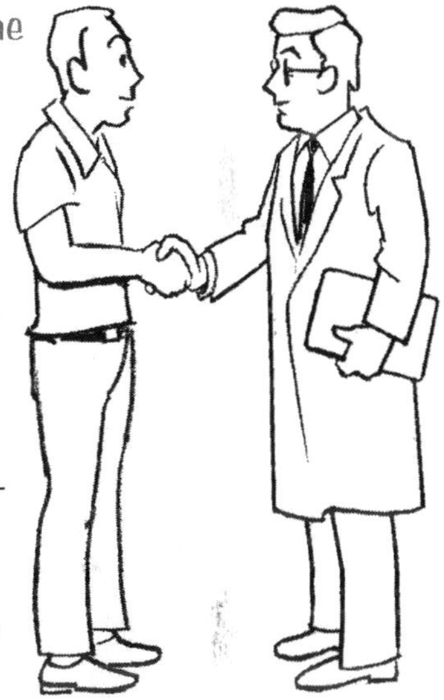

The following forms are samples of what the authors use in their private practices. They were created from many sources and will probably need to be heavily modified for use in other practices. These will be available in a downloadable form from our website. There are several forms not included here. Often this is because they are legal documents that may be drastically different between states. Others are absolutely necessary, but are often provided by insurance companies and practitioners must use the provided forms. The following is a list of these, though the list may not be complete.

It can be helpful to have forms numbered with a master notebook as well as a digital folder of these as well. This notebook and folder has all your forms in order and a master list of the forms in the front. It is also a very good idea to have the date each form was created or changed in an inconspicuous space, so that employees always know what is the latest version of the form.

Informed consent

This is a necessary form that *all* patients must sign before *any* treatment is provided. It basically says what the provider does and what could go wrong. *All* medical procedures need to have a signed informed consent. It is not just required for protection and malpractice, but it is highly unethical to perform a medical procedure without explaining it to a patient and allowing them to say no. Generally, malpractice insurance companies provide accepted informed consent forms. If you are insured by the American Acupuncture Council [AAC], for example, the informed consent is on the opposite side of the arbitration agreement. Always make sure these forms are signed before initiating treatment. It is considered an ethical violation of a patient's autonomy, and is probably illegal, to perform a medical procedure without an informed consent.

Notice of health information privacy practices

This is required under HIPAA. While there are some standard versions, a provider should find an appropriate version and modify it for their practice.

Report of findings

A report of findings is a form filled out at the end of the first visit or sometimes the beginning of their second visit. It outlines what the practitioner found in his or her history and examination, the diagnosis and the treatment plan. Many experts believe this is an extremely important form for patient retention and practice building when fully explained to the patient.

New patient checklist

One of the most helpful forms in maintaining an orderly office and making sure all paperwork is properly filled out and in the patient's file is a new patient checklist. It should be the first thing visible in the administrative portion of a patient's file. All the items listed on this form should be completed before treating the patient. Following are two different examples of this form.

New Patient Checklist

Patient Name:________________________ Date ________________

- ❑ Form 103 – New Patient Information
- ❑ Generate Patient Number, 2 last name initials, first initial, 2 digit year, and 2 digit month ______________________________
- ❑ Form 105 – Informed Consent
- ❑ Form 107 – Patient Care Financial Agreement
- ❑ Form 109 – Notice of Health Information Privacy Practices
- ❑ Please make a copy of patient's official ID, such as a drivers license
- ❑ Add as new patient to Office Ally or medical software program
- ❑ Add to MyReceptionist or Other
- ❑ Add to mailing list
- ❑ Make folder with Patient Label
- ❑ If patient has allergies, place appropriate sticker on outside of patient folder
- ❑ If patient has a blood borne or contagious disease, place appropriate sticker on outside of patient folder
- ❑ Send a welcome card
- ❑ Send a thank you card to referrer, if referred

Plus, If Insurance patient:

- ❑ Copy of Insurance card, both sides
- ❑ From 201 – Insurance Verification **Please do immediately**
- ❑ Form 203 – Assignment of Benefits
- ❑ If ASH patient, Form 225 – ASH Member Billing Acknowledgement

NEW PATIENT CHECKLIST

Patient: Date:

Copy of Drivers License in file

Insurance Verified w/verification form in the file and info in the computer (notes). If ASH, verified on-line & Printed copy on file

Verify that a new patient evaluation was charged in the patients account

Check info put into computer:

***** Always open a cash case first, then add a case (INS/WC/PI, etc) if needed *****

PERSONAL screen
- -all personal info
- -referral source

CASE screen
- -description of case
- -Assign provider
- -Managed care profile set
- -Edit Comments if necessary (put Rx Exp info, co-pay amt, etc.)

GUARANTOR screen
- -Set guarantor 1info (if new, click new)
- -copy patient info

POLICY & COVERAGE (**INS, PI or WC ONLY**)
- -assign payor
- -Set responsibility to payor % coverage, set to 100%
- -Enter policy ID (ID off ins card OR claim #)
- -Enter group # for ins (not WC or PI)
- ___ Enter the effective date of coverage (WC or PI is date of injury)
- -ASHP only, must enter: group #, effective date of coverage, group name (HealthNet, ex)

CONDITION screen
- - Don't worry about Diagnosis - Billing Manager will do
- ___ If WC or PI, check appropriate box
- ___ Illness/Injury occurred date: WC and PI is the date of injury if it is insurance or cash, enter the first date they are coming in
- - Primary Guarantor set

NOTES screen - Make sure to enter INSURANCE VERIFICATION information

1. _______ Color dot to match case
2. _______ Verify that Thank You Card was sent
3. _______ Verify that REFERRAL CARD was sent
4. _______ If pt has BLUE CROSS/BLUE SHIELD or ASHP was the correct Fee Increase form signed? If AETNA, Was benefits acknowledgment form signed? (Acu only)
5. _______ If the patient has a P.O.S. Ins Plan, have you added "Process out of Network" to HCFA space avail. in Edit Comments/CASE tab?
6. _______ Does an ASHP Intake Form need to be swapped with original? - Please give to practitioner to rewrite.
7. _______ Check Intake form for BLOOD DISORDERS, HEPATITS, HIV +, INFECTIOUS DISEASES – If any are (+), Add addt'l Biohazrd sticker to left inside cover of file along crease
8. _______ FOR MINORS – Did we get the "Consent to treat Minor" form signed?

Completed by:

New patient information forms

A form of this type is not only absolutely imperative for proper administration of patients, it is illegal to treat without it. While most practitioners believe Asian medicine is safe, and it is, there are definitely issues with practice. To initiate treatment without knowing if there are any contraindications or concerns (such as pregnancy, pharmaceuticals, hemophilia, etc.), would be considered medical negligence and can result in getting sued or losing one's license.

This is a confidential questionnaire designed to help us determine the best treatment plan for you. If you have any questions, please ask. Thank you.

Personal Information

Date ______________

Name ______________________________________

Birthdate ______________ Sex: ☐ Male ☐ Female

Social Security Number ________________________

Marital status: ☐ Married ☐ Single ☐ Other Number of children________

Home Address ______________________________________

City ______________________ State _____ Zip ______________

Home Ph. ______________ Work Ph.______________ Cell Ph./Other______________

Occupation ______________________________________

Email address ______________________________________

Is it okay to send you announcements and appointment reminders through email? ☐ Yes ☐ No

Emergency Contact ________________________ Relationship________________

Phone ______________ ☐ Home ☐ Work ☐ Cell

Who can we thank for referring you to this office? ______________________________

How did you hear about us? ☐ Friend ☐ Brochure ☐ Other______________________

Have you received acupuncture or herbal therapy before?

☐ Herbs ☐ Acupuncture ☐ Both ☐ Neither

FOR OFFICE USE ONLY

Medical Record #____________

Form 103 Revision Date: 4/18/08

What are the main health problems for which you are seeking treatment?

Clinical notes (Practitioner use)

____

____

____

____

Please list any other problems you currently have

____

____

____

____

Please list any allergies, food sensitivities, or food cravings that you have..

____

____

____

Please list any accidents, surgeries or hospitalizations (include dates).

____

____

____

____

____

On the following chart please indicate any illnesses you (please include date) or your family members have had. ***All Information is Confidential.***

Illness	You (date)	Family	Illness	You (Date)	Family
Cancer			Diabetes		
Emotional Disorders			Hepatitis		
Heart Diseases			High Blood Pressure		
Infectious Diseases			Rheumatic Fever		
Seizures			Stroke		
Sexually Transmitted Diseases			Other ________		

Please list any medications you are currently taking and why:

____

____

Please list any vitamins, supplements, and herbs you are currently taking and why:

____

____

Substance	Never	Infrequently	Once a week	A few times a week	Once a day	Twice a Day	More than twice a day
Tobacco							
Coffee or Black Tea							
Soda							
Alcohol							
Non-medical drugs							
Exercise							

How do you feel about the following areas of your life? Please check the appropriate box and indicate any problems you may be experiencing.

	Great	Good	Fair	Poor	Bad	Your Comments
Spouse or Significant other						
Family						
Diet						
Sex						
Self						
Work						

Symptom Survey

The following is a list of symptoms. Please put a plus (+) sign if you frequently experience the symptom, a minus (-) sign if you sometimes experience it, or leave it blank if you never experience it.

Lack of appetite	
Excessive appetite	
Loose stool or diarrhea	
Digestion problems, indigestion	
Vomiting	
Belching, burping	
Heartburn	
Feeling of retention of food in stomach	
Tendency to become obsessive in work, relationships	
Insomnia, difficulty sleeping	
Heart palpitations	
Cold hands and feet	
Nightmares	
Mentally restless	
Laughing for no apparent reason	
Angina pains	
Abdominal Pain	
Chest pain	
Sciatic Pain	
Headaches	

Cough	
Shortness of breath	
Decreased sense of smell	
Nasal problems	
Skin problems	
Feeling of claustrophobia	
Bronchitis	
Colitis or diverticulitis	
Constipation	
Hemorrhoids	
Recent use of antibiotics	
Eye problems	
Jaundice (yellowish eyes or skin)	
Hepatitis	
Difficulty digesting oily foods	
Gall stones	
Light colored stool	
Soft or brittle nails	
Easily angered or agitated	
Difficulty in making plans or decisions	
Spasms or twitching of muscles	

Low back pain	
Knee problems	
Hearing impairment	
Ear ringing (Tinnitus)	
Kidney stones	
Decreased sex drive	
Hair loss	
Urinary problems	
Fatigue	
Edema	
Blood in stool	
Black tarry stool	
Easily bruised	
Difficulty stopping bleeding	
Asthma	
Tendency to catch colds easily	
Intolerance to weather changes	
Allergies	
Hay fever	
Dizziness	
Tendency to faint easily	
High blood pressure	
High cholesterol levels	
Sudden weight loss	

For Men:	
Prostate problems	
Painful or burning urination	
Pain or coldness in the genital region	
Other	

For Women:		
Are you pregnant?		Last OB/GYN Exam:
Pre-menstrual pain or discomfort		Results:
Menstrual pain or discomfort		
Irregular menstrual cycle		Other:
Swelling or pain in breasts		

Personal injury Questionnaire

This form should be filled out upon initiating a personal injury case.

Personal Injury Questionnaire

Name ______________________ Phone# (   ) ______________________

Address ______________________ City ____________ State ______ Zip ________

Age ______ Birth Date ____________ Sex ______ SS# ______________________

Employer's Name ______________________ Email Address ______________

Your Auto Insurance ____________ Policy# ____________ Claim# ____________

Name on Policy (if other than self) ______________________

Your Adjuster's Name ______________________ Adjuster Phone# ______________

Responsible Party's Name ______________________

Responsible Party's Insurance Co. ______________________ Phone# (   ) ____________

Is third party accepting liability? (circle) Yes No Not sure

ATTORNEY

Name ______________________ Phone# (   ) ______________________

Address ______________________ City ____________ State ______ Zip ________

NATURE OF ACCIDENT

1. Date of Accident ______________________ Time of Day ______________ am/pm
2. Were you: ❑ Driver ❑ Passenger ❑ Front Seat ❑ Back Seat
3. Number of people in your vehicle ________ Were you wearing a seatbelt? (circle) Yes No
4. What direction were you headed? ❑ North ❑ South ❑ East ❑ West
   on (name of street) ______________________
5. What direction was the other vehicle traveling? ❑ North ❑ South ❑ East ❑ West
   on (name of street) ______________________
6. Were you struck from: ❑ Behind ❑ Front ❑ Left side ❑ Right side
7. Approximate speed of your vehicle ____________ mph Other Vehicle ____________ mph
8. Were you knocked unconscious? (circle) Yes No If yes, for how long? ____________
9. Were the police notified? (circle) Yes No

9a. Do you have a police report? (circle) Yes No If yes, please provide a copy.

10. In your own words, please describe the accident:

____

____

____

continued on the next page

11. Did you have any physical complaints BEFORE THE ACCIDENT? (circle) Yes No If yes, please describe in detail:

____

12. Please describe how you felt:
    a. DURING the accident: _______________
    b. IMMEDIATELY AFTER the accident: _______________
    c. LATER THAT DAY: _______________
    d. THE NEXT DAY: _______________

13. What are your PRESENT complaints and symptoms? _______________

14. Do you have any congenital (from birth) factors that relate to this problem? (circle) Yes No If yes, please describe in detail: _______________

15. Do you have any previous illness that relates to this case? (circle) Yes No If yes, please describe in detail:

____

16. Have you ever been involved in an accident before? (circle) Yes No If yes, please describe, including date(s) and type(s) of accident(s), as well as injury(ies) received : _______________

17. Where were you taken after this accident? _______________

18. Have you been treated by another doctor since the accident? (circle) Yes No If yes, please list the doctor's name and address _______________

18a. What type of treatment did you receive? _______________

19. Since this injury occured, are your symptoms: ❑ Improving ❑ Getting worse ❑ Same

20. Check the symptoms you have noticed since the accident:

❑ Headache	❑ Irritability	❑ Numbness in Toes	❑ Face Flushed	❑ Feel Cold
❑ Neck Pain	❑ Chest Pain	❑ Shortness of Breath	❑ Buzzing in Eyes	❑ Hands Cold
❑ Neck Stiff	❑ Dizziness	❑ Fatigue	❑ Loss of Balance	❑ Stomach Upset
❑ Sleeping Problems	❑ Head Seems Too Heavy	❑ Depression	❑ Fainting	❑ Constipation
❑ Back Pain	❑ Pins & Needles in Arms	❑ Lights Bother Eyes	❑ Loss of Smell	❑ Cold Sweats
❑ Nervousness	❑ Pins & Needles in Legs	❑ Loss of Memory	❑ Loss of Taste	❑ Fever
❑ Tension	❑ Numbness in Fingers	❑ Ears Ring	❑ Diarrhea	❑ ________

Symptoms other than above: _______________

21. Have you lost time from work as a result of this accident? (circle) Yes No If yes, please complete this question.
    a. Last day worked _______________
    b. Type of employment _______________

22. Do you notice any activity restrictions as a result of this injury? (circle) Yes No If yes, please describe in detail: _______________

22a. Are there any job duties that agravate your condition? (circle) Yes No If yes, please describe in detail:

____

Patient Signature _______________ Date _______________

Super bill

A super bill is used when a patient is going to be sending in the bill for reimbursement from a third party. Some offices use them to keep track of what treatments have been administered. These are not absolutely necessary. Filling out a CMS-1500 form and giving it to the patient is just as good, but super bills are easier to use.

Many patients have HRAs and HSAs that reimburse them for their medical bills. When a patient submits for reimbursement, the receipt or super bill must include:

- the providers name, address, and Tax ID or Social Security Number
- the ICD (diagnosis) code must be listed
- the CPT (treatment) codes must also be listed
- The amount the patient paid must also be included.

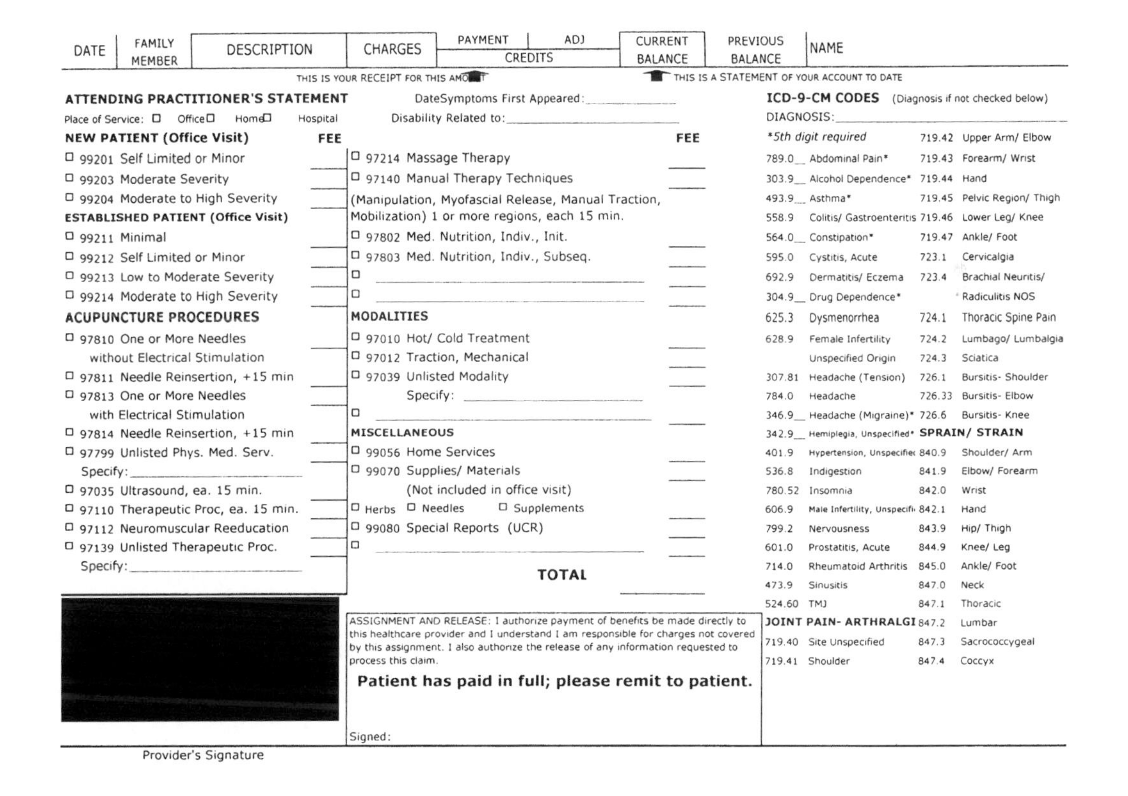

DATE	FAMILY MEMBER	DESCRIPTION	CHARGES	PAYMENT (CREDITS)	ADJ (CREDITS)	CURRENT BALANCE	PREVIOUS BALANCE	NAME

THIS IS YOUR RECEIPT FOR THIS AMOUNT — THIS IS A STATEMENT OF YOUR ACCOUNT TO DATE

ATTENDING PRACTITIONER'S STATEMENT

Place of Service: ☐ Office☐ Home☐ Hospital

DateSymptoms First Appeared:____________

Disability Related to:____________

NEW PATIENT (Office Visit) FEE
- ☐ 99201 Self Limited or Minor ____
- ☐ 99203 Moderate Severity ____
- ☐ 99204 Moderate to High Severity ____

ESTABLISHED PATIENT (Office Visit)
- ☐ 99211 Minimal ____
- ☐ 99212 Self Limited or Minor ____
- ☐ 99213 Low to Moderate Severity ____
- ☐ 99214 Moderate to High Severity ____

ACUPUNCTURE PROCEDURES
- ☐ 97810 One or More Needles without Electrical Stimulation ____
- ☐ 97811 Needle Reinsertion, +15 min ____
- ☐ 97813 One or More Needles with Electrical Stimulation ____
- ☐ 97814 Needle Reinsertion, +15 min ____
- ☐ 97799 Unlisted Phys. Med. Serv. Specify:____________ ____
- ☐ 97035 Ultrasound, ea. 15 min. ____
- ☐ 97110 Therapeutic Proc, ea. 15 min. ____
- ☐ 97112 Neuromuscular Reeducation ____
- ☐ 97139 Unlisted Therapeutic Proc. Specify:____________ ____

FEE
- ☐ 97214 Massage Therapy ____
- ☐ 97140 Manual Therapy Techniques ____

(Manipulation, Myofascial Release, Manual Traction, Mobilization) 1 or more regions, each 15 min.
- ☐ 97802 Med. Nutrition, Indiv., Init. ____
- ☐ 97803 Med. Nutrition, Indiv., Subseq. ____
- ☐ ____________ ____
- ☐ ____________ ____

MODALITIES
- ☐ 97010 Hot/ Cold Treatment ____
- ☐ 97012 Traction, Mechanical ____
- ☐ 97039 Unlisted Modality Specify: ____________ ____
- ☐ ____________ ____

MISCELLANEOUS
- ☐ 99056 Home Services ____
- ☐ 99070 Supplies/ Materials (Not included in office visit) ____
- ☐ Herbs ☐ Needles ☐ Supplements
- ☐ 99080 Special Reports (UCR) ____
- ☐ ____________ ____

TOTAL ____

ICD-9-CM CODES (Diagnosis if not checked below)

DIAGNOSIS:____________

*5th digit required

Code	Diagnosis	Code	Diagnosis
789.0__	Abdominal Pain*	719.42	Upper Arm/ Elbow
303.9__	Alcohol Dependence*	719.43	Forearm/ Wrist
493.9__	Asthma*	719.44	Hand
558.9	Colitis/ Gastroenteritis	719.45	Pelvic Region/ Thigh
564.0__	Constipation*	719.46	Lower Leg/ Knee
595.0	Cystitis, Acute	719.47	Ankle/ Foot
692.9	Dermatitis/ Eczema	723.1	Cervicalgia
304.9__	Drug Dependence*	723.4	Brachial Neuritis/ Radiculitis NOS
625.3	Dysmenorrhea	724.1	Thoracic Spine Pain
628.9	Female Infertility Unspecified Origin	724.2	Lumbago/ Lumbalgia
307.81	Headache (Tension)	724.3	Sciatica
784.0	Headache	726.1	Bursitis- Shoulder
346.9__	Headache (Migraine)*	726.33	Bursitis- Elbow
342.9__	Hemiplegia, Unspecified*	726.6	Bursitis- Knee
401.9	Hypertension, Unspecified	**SPRAIN/ STRAIN**	
536.8	Indigestion	840.9	Shoulder/ Arm
780.52	Insomnia	841.9	Elbow/ Forearm
606.9	Male Infertility, Unspecified	842.0	Wrist
799.2	Nervousness	842.1	Hand
601.0	Prostatitis, Acute	843.9	Hip/ Thigh
714.0	Rheumatoid Arthritis	844.9	Knee/ Leg
473.9	Sinusitis	845.0	Ankle/ Foot
524.60	TMJ	847.0	Neck
JOINT PAIN- ARTHRALGI		847.1	Thoracic
719.40	Site Unspecified	847.2	Lumbar
719.41	Shoulder	847.3	Sacrococcygeal
		847.4	Coccyx

ASSIGNMENT AND RELEASE: I authorize payment of benefits be made directly to this healthcare provider and I understand I am responsible for charges not covered by this assignment. I also authorize the release of any information requested to process this claim.

Patient has paid in full; please remit to patient.

Signed:

Provider's Signature

Patient care financial agreement

The patient care financial agreement helps lay out a patient's financial responsibilities. It is a legal agreement and should be run past a lawyer to be sure there are not any issues. It should be handed out with the fee schedule and, if the patient is from American Specialty Health, the form outlining what is covered and what is not. Some patients feel asking for a credit card is very heavy-handed and it is up the practitioner whether or not to include it. In addition, a patient's driver's license should be photocopied and kept with this form.

Patient Care Financial Agreement

Dear Patient,

We want you to have a clear understanding of our policy concerning payment and insurance. Our office accepts cash, checks, American Express, Visa, MasterCard, and Discover cards.

If you have NO INSURANCE you will need to pay your charges in full on each visit.

If you have HEALTH INSURANCE:

Please bear in mind that you are ultimately responsible for payment of your charges in full.

On each visit, you will need to pay the estimated percentage of your charges not covered by your insurance.

We will notify you of any amounts your insurance fails to pay within sixty (60) days. You will have another thirty (30) days to call your insurance company. Any amount owing over ninety (90) days by your insurance company will be charged to your credit card.

Any insurance checks you might receive are to be brought to our office promptly. If you fail to do so within one week of receiving it, the check amount will be billed to your credit card.

Insurance companies do not always pay for every procedure performed. You are responsible for any procedures not covered by your insurance. This may include massage, moxibustion, cupping, and gua sha among other procedures. Herbs are rarely covered by insurance. Any amount not covered by your insurance must be paid within thirty (30) days of your being notified of the amount. Amounts owed over thirty (30) days will be charged to your credit card.

I hereby authorize New Life Health Partners or its agents/employees to bill my credit card for amounts unpaid by insurance as specified above.

□ Mastercard □ Amex □ Visa □ Discover

Print name as it appears on credit card: ______________________________

Card Number: ______________________ Expiration Date: ____________

Signature: ___________________________ Date: ____________

Form 107, Rev. 4/18/08

Assignment of benefits form

The assignment of benefits form is another necessary form when billing insurance. Without it, the insurance company must send the reimbursement checks to the patient, not the practitioner. This either confuses the patient or creates a need for debt collection. Neither are desirable when accepting insurance. A practitioner needs to put "signature on file" in boxes 12 & 13 of the CMS 1500 form (the universal

AUTHORIZATION AND ASSIGNMENT OF BENEFITS TO PRACTITIONER

Patient's Name ______________ Social Security Number ______________

Insured's name (if different) ______________

1. I authorize the release of any information concerning my health to any insurance company, attorney, or adjuster as necessary to process any claim for payment for any practitioner working for [Company] incurred by me. I also authorize the insurance company to furnish to the clinic named above, any information regarding my claims under the policy of the Social Security Act.

2. In consideration of any practitioner working for [Company] rendering of treatment to me without immediate compensation, I therefore authorize and irrevocably assign my right to payment of the bill from any insurance company providing coverage to me for such expenses.

3. With reference to any contracted insurance company providing coverage to me for medical care and treatment, I understand, authorize, and agree that no payments due me under said contract shall be made to me for any other medical expenses incurred until [Company's] bill for all medical care and treatment is paid in full

4. In the event any insurance company obligated by contractual agreement to make payments to me or to the practitioner refuses to make such payments upon demand, I hereby irrevocably assign and transfer to the practitioner any cause of action that exists in my favor against any such company, and authorize the practitioner to prosecute that action either in my name or in his name and further to compromise, settle, or otherwise resolve said claim.

5. I hereby appoint the practitioner, and any of his duly authorized agents and employees, to endorse any and all checks, drafts, or money orders which are made payable to the undersigned for medical services or the like which have been, or are to be, performed by the practitioner.

Notice to insurance company of assignment:
You are instructed to pay directly to the practitioner at this office for all professional services rendered to me . This instruction to you is an assignment of my rights under the medical coverage of the insurance policy. Any sum of money paid under this assignment shall be credited-to my account.

A photocopy of this Assignment shall be considered as effective and valid as the original.

I also authorize the release of any information pertinent to my case to any insurance company, adjuster, or attorney involved in this case.

Dated at ____________ this ____________ day of ____________ 20 ______

______________ Patient's Signature

______________ Witness

______________ Insured's Signature (If different or required)

Form 203, Rev. 4/14/08

insurance submission form) in order to receive the check from the insurance company. Legally, they can only do so if the patient signed an assignment of benefits form. Again, this is a legal form and it may be wise to show it to an attorney.

Assignment and Instruction for Direct Payment to Doctor

Patient Name:
Insurance Company:

I hereby instruct the above name insurance company to pay be check made out to and mailed directly to:

[Insert your name, address, and phone # here]

for professional medical expense benefits allowable, and otherwise payable to me under my current insurance policy or by a 3rd party payor who would otherwise pay me directly, as payment toward the total charges for professional services rendered.

THIS IS A DIRECT ASSIGNMENT OF MY RIGHTS AND BENEFITS UNDER THIS POLICY AND/OR CLAIM.

This payment will not exceed my indebtedness to the above-mentioned assignee, and I have agreed to pay, in a current manner, any balance of said professional fees for non-covered servics and/or fees, over and above the insurance payment or as required by the insurance policy. I also authorize the release of any information pertinent to my case to any insurance company, adjuster, or attorney for the purpose of securing payment under this policy of insurance.

Date:
Signature of Policy Holder or Claimant:

Insurance verification forms

There are three basic insurance verification forms: the basic one for most insurances, a personal injury verification, and a workers compensation verification. Following are examples of each.

Date received:

INSURANCE VERIFICATION

Patient: ____________________________ Insured ID# ______________________DOB:_________

Insurance Co., Tel# ____

ACUPUNCTURE BENEFITS PROVIDER: _______________ IN/OUT OF NETWORK? _________

[YOUR NAME OR BIZ NAME HERE]: ____

YOUR TAX ID#: ___________________________ NPI#: _______________________________

If you are out of network, use the patient's SS# to check benefits.

MD coverage only? YES/NO (If yes, and you are connected to an MD's office, use that Tax ID and NPI for billing purposes)

Are there ACU benefits? _________ Are there Discount Programs? ____________________

What type of policy (HMO, PPO, HRA): ________ Is a referral required? __________

If AETNA, is acu covered in lieu of anesthesia only? Yes/No For nausea only? Yes/No

Under ptx group#, are ICD codes 346.01 (migraine) and 724.2 (chronic lumbago) covered?

Are CPT Codes 97810 and 97811 covered? Yes/No

Any other coverage notes or specifics? ____

Effective dates of coverage____________________ Group# __________________

Is coverage Calendar Year or Other: ________ Primary or Secondary Ins? (Circle)

Deductible? How much? ___________ How much met so far? _______

Coverage Info and/or Co-pay, etc.: ______________________ Copay set by TA: ________

visits per yr or visit $ max per yr __________ How many/much used? _____ Max'd? ____

Out of pocket maximum: _________ Is Acu combined with any other service? _________

If MD only: Are physician office visits covered? ______ Max per year: __________

Time Frame to submit claims: ____

Claims Address: ____

Other claims / Eclipse ? Coverage Notes:

____

Note if anything needs to be sent with claims, i.e., Letter of Med. necessity, certification, notes, etc.

Verfied by: _____ Date: ________ Spoke to: ________________________ Ref. #: ______________

PERSONAL INJURY INSURANCE VERIFICATION

Today's Date: ______________

Patient's Name: ______________________________

Claim #: ______________________________

Date of Injury (DOI): ______________________________

Patient's Auto Insurance Co.: ______________________________

Adjuster's Name: ______________________________

Tel #: ______________________ Ext.: __________

Fax #: ______________________

Is there med-pay coverage? ______________________________**

If yes, how much? ______________________________

If yes, is it excess to their primary health insurance? ______________________

Address to send claims: ______________________________

____

Are chart notes required?: ______________________________

If yes, how often: ______________________________

Name & number of customer service agent spoken to:

____

____

Attorney name and contact information: ______________________

____

Verified by: ______________________________

**If the patient does not have med-pay, you will need to see if the patient has regular health insurance coverage. Additionally, you will need to get a signed lien from the patient's attorney (have the patient sign one even if they do not yet have an attorney and keep it on file). Remember–3rd party liens are highly discouraged–they are a huge gamble.

Workers' Compensation Insurance Verification

Today's Date: ____________

Patient's Name: ______________________________

Claim #: ___________________________________

Date of Injury (DOI): _________________________

Insurance Co.: _______________________________

Adjuster's Name: _____________________________

Tel #: ______________________ Ext.: __________

Fax #: ______________________

Utilization reviewer (UR) Name: ___________________________

Tel #: ______________________ Ext.: __________

Fax #: ______________________

Has the claim been approved? ______ Is the claim open and active?

____

Address to send claims: ____

____

Are chart notes required?: _____________________________________

If yes, how often: ____

Attorney name and contact information: ____________________________

____

Verified by: ___________________________

Credit Authorization Form

This form is used when one party would like to pay for another party's treatments.

Credit Authorization Form

This agreement is for the undersigned to pay for another patient's medical care provided by New Life Health Partners.

The undersigned agrees to pay for (☐ ____________ number of visits **or** ☐ unlimited visits)

The undersigned agrees to pay for herbs for this patient: ☐ Yes ☐ No

This agreement is valid until ____________(date).

I hereby authorize New Life Health Partners or its agents/employees to bill my credit card within the specified parameters above.

☐ MasterCard ☐ Amex ☐ Visa ☐ Discover

Date: ____________

Print name as it appears on credit card: ______________________________

Credit Card Number: ______________________ Expiration Date: ____________

Signature: ______________________

Form 611, Rev. 6/23/08

Personal Injury Payment Acceptance Policy Letter

This letter is a very useful explanation of the process of a personal injury claim and why the practitioner needs all the information requested.

Personal Injury Payment Acceptance Policy Sample Letter

Dear Patient,

If you have been involved in an automobile accident, we will need a copy of your car insurance card. We will then verify if you have medical payments as part of your coverage. If you do, we will bill your car insurance for your care. If you were a passenger in someone else's car, we will need a copy of the driver's car insurance to see if they have medical payments coverage for you.

You (or the driver) pay for this benefit and it *does not* increase your premiums.

Your insurance will be reimbursed from the responsible party's insurance upon settlement of the claim. If you were at fault, your auto insurance simply pays your bills with no reimbursement to them.

If you were hit by an uninsured motorist and you have uninsured motorist coverage, your insurance will pay for your care at the conclusion of treatment.

If you do not have medical payments coverage, or health insurance, you will need to get an attorney. This both protects you and the doctor. If you need a referral to an attorney, we will be happy to refer you to a few that we work with.

This office does *not* accept third party liens. A third party lien is a type of case where the other party (insurance of the person who hit you) accepts responsibility for your medical care, but *does not* pay us directly. They typically refuse to pay us directly citing that their responsibility is to you, the person their insured hit, not to all of the providers you saw. Since we are unable to secure a direct method of payment, we do not accept these circumstances.

As with any case, if we are unable to secure payment from the auto insurance, attorney, health insurance, etc., or they have failed to make full payment and a balance is owing, you understand that you are ultimately responsible for payment of your case out of any settlements that you receive or otherwise.

I have read and understand the Personal Injury policies of Successful Acupuncture clinic.

Print Patient Name________________________Date____________

____

Patient Signature

NOTICE OF ATTORNEY LIEN (SAMPLE)

TO: Attorney
FROM:
RE: Medical Reports and Practitioner's Lien DOI:

I do hereby authorize the above Practitioner to furnish you, my Attorney, with a full report of his examination, diagnosis, treatment, prognosis, etc. of myself in regard to the accident in which I was recently involved.

I hereby authorize and direct you, my Attorney, to pay to said Practitioner such sums as may be due and owing him for medical service rendered me by reason of this accident and by reason of any other bills that are due his office and to withhold such sums from any settlement, judgment, or verdict as may be necessary to adequately protect said Practitioner.

And I hereby further give a lien on my case to said Practitioner against any and all proceeds of any settlement, judgment or verdict which may be paid to you, my Attorney, or myself as the result of the injuries for which I have been treated or injuries in connection herewith.

I agree never to rescind this document and that a rescission will not be honored by my Attorney. I hereby instruct that in the event another Attorney is substituted in this matter, the new Attorney honor this lien as inherent to the settlement and enforceable upon the case as if it were executed by him.

I fully understand that I am directly and fully responsible to said Practitioner for all medical benefits submitted by him for service rendered me and that this agreement is made solely for said Practitioner's additional protection. I further understand that such payment is not contingent on any settlement, judgment or verdict by which I may eventually recover said fee. If this account is assigned for collection and/or suit, collection costs and/or interest, and/or Attorney fees, and/or court costs will be added to the total amount due.

Please acknowledge this letter by signing below and returning to Practitioner's office. I have been advised that if my Attorney does not wish to await payment but may declare the entire balance due and payable. Also, upon settlement of this case, I instruct you, my Attorney, to provide said Practitioner all medical records, billing from other providers, settlement amounts from insurance companies and third-party individuals and the proposed settlement split between all parties, upon their request. This information will be used solely for the purpose of the settlement negotiation for this case.

Dated: ______________________________

Patient's Signature: ______________________________

Witness: ______________________________

Print Patient's Name: ______________________________

ACKNOWLEDGEMENT OF ATTORNEY

The undersigned being Attorney of record for the above patient does hereby agree to observe all the terms of the above and agrees to withhold such sums from any settlement, judgment or verdict as may be necessary to adequately protect said Practitioner above named. Any settlement of this claim without honoring this assignment/lien will cause you to be responsible to this office for payment. The prevailing party in any litigation resulting from enforcement of this lien shall be entitled to actual Attorney's fees and court costs.

Dated: ______________________________

Attorney's Signature: ______________________________

Attorney: Please date, sign and return one copy to above Practitioner's office at once.

—Keep one copy for your records—

This form is used for personal injury (PI) cases. The patient must sign it and you must have their attorney sign it (always keep the original). Only with this lien signed and completed will your bills be paid from the final PI settlement.

Summary of Notice of Privacy Practices

HIPAA requires a Notice of Privacy practices that is available to any patient. This summary is a nice handout to give to a patient. It does not, however, replace the full Notice of Privacy Practices.

*****FOR PATIENT TO KEEP*****

Summary of Notice of Privacy Practices

A new federal law known as the Health Insurance Portability and Accountability Act of 1996 ("HIPAA") went into force on April 14, 2003. We are required to give you a printed copy of our Notice of Privacy Practices. For your convenience, we are providing this brief summary. Each section has a corresponding section in our full Notice, which we encourage you to read in its entirety. We are required to ask you to sign a one-time acknowledgment that you have received our full Notice. We will provide you with a complete copy of our Notice of Privacy Practices if you so desire.

Your rights as a patient. You have many new and important rights with respect to your protected health information. These are summarized below and described in detail in our full Notice of Privacy Practices.

Use of Protected Health Information. We are permitted to use your protected health information for treatment purposes, to facilitate our being paid, and to conduct our business and evaluate the quality and efficiency of our processes. Also, we are permitted to disclose protected health information under specific circumstances to other entities. We have put into place safeguards to protect the privacy of your health information. However, there may be incidental disclosures of limited information, such as overhearing a conversation, that occur in the course of authorized communications, routine treatment, payment, or the operations of our practice. HIPAA recognizes that such disclosures may be extremely difficult to avoid entirely, and considers them as permissible.

For entities that are not covered under HIPAA to which we must send protected health information for treatment, payment, or operational purposes, we require that they sign a contract in which they agree to protect the confidentiality of this information.

Disclosure of Protected Health Information Requiring Your Authorization. For disclosures that are not related to treatment, payment, or operations, we will obtain your specific written consent, except as described below.

Disclosure of Protected Health Information Not Requiring Your Authorization. We are required by state and federal law to make disclosures of certain protected health information without obtaining your authorization. Examples include mandated reporting of conditions affecting public health, subpoenas, and other legal requests.

Communication to You of Confidential Information by Alternative Means. If you make a written request, we will communicate confidential information to you by reasonable alternative means, or to an alternative address.

Restrictions to Use and Disclosure. You may request restrictions to the use or disclosure of your protected health information, but we are not required by HIPAA to agree to such requests. However, if we do agree, then we are bound to honor your request. In the course of our use and disclosure of your protected health information, only the minimum amount of such information will be used to accomplish the intended goal.

Access to Protected Health Information. You may request access to or a copy of your medical records in writing. We will provide these within the time period specified, unless we are forbidden under HIPAA or by applicable state law to provide such records. If we deny access, we will tell you why. You may appeal this decision, which, under specified circumstances, will be reviewed by a third party not involved in the denial.

Amendments to Medical Records. You may request in writing that corrections be made to your medical records. We will either accept the amendments, and notify appropriate parties, or deny your request with an explanation. You have rights to dispute such denials and have your objections noted in your medical record.

Accounting of disclosures of Protected Health Information. You may request in writing an accounting of disclosures of your protected health information. This accounting excludes disclosures made in the course of treatment, payment, or operations, and disclosures that were made as a result of your written authorization.

Other Uses of Your Health Information. Optional uses, as permitted under HIPAA, are listed in our complete Notice of Privacy Practices.

How to Lodge Complaints Related to Perceived Violations of Your Privacy Rights. You may register a complaint about any of our privacy practices with our Privacy Official or with the Secretary of Health and Human Services without fear of retaliation, coercion, or intimidation.

Acknowledgment of Receipt of Notice of Privacy Practices

According to HIPAA, every patient needs to sign this form, acknowledging they have received a copy of the practice's privacy practices.

Use and disclosure of protected health information is regulated by a federal law known as 'The Health Insurance Portability and Accountability Act of 1996' (HIPPA). Under HIPPA, providers of healthcare are required to give patients their Notice of Privacy Practices for Protected Health Information and make a good faith effort to obtain a written acknowledgment that this notice was received.

Therefore, I, ______________________________ (printed name of patient or personal representative), acknowledge that, ______________ (your business name) has provided a written copy of its Notice of Privacy Practices for Protected Heath Information to (check one) ___myself or ___ specify:

(If signing as a personal representative, documentation of your legal right to do so must be provided.)

Signature of Patient or Personal Representative

Date (mm/22/yyyy)

Printed Name

Relationship to patient (if not self)

To be completed by

___ We made a good faith attempt to provide the above named patient with a copy of our Notice of Privacy Practices for protected Health Information, but we were not successful for the following reasons:

Printed name	Title	Signature	Date (mm/dd/yyyy)

Appendix C: Glossary

AAC: American Acupuncture Council. A malpractice insurance provider for acupuncturists.

ABC: See Advanced Billing Concepts.

Accounts receivables (AR): This is an accounting term that refers to money that is owed the business, for example insurance reimbursements.

ACOEM: See American College of Occupational and Environmental Medicine.

Adjuster: See insurance adjuster.

ADLs: Activities of daily living. These are important to note in chart notes and refer to whether the patient can accomplish basic activities such as buttoning a shirt or opening a can.

Advanced billing concepts (ABC): This is an alternative coding system for current practices in alternative medicine, nursing and integrative healthcare. They are not widely used or accepted and Current Procedural Terminology (CPT) codes should be used as they are the standard.

Allowed amount: This is the amount a contracted provider has agreed to receive for a specific medical procedure. In-network providers are contractually prevented from pursuing patients for any more than this amount. This becomes probably the biggest advantage of out-of-network providers: they can pursue patients for more than the allowed amount.

Alternative Link, Inc.: The company that created the ABC coding system

AMA: American Medical Association.

American College of Occupational and Environmental Medicine (ACOEM): Their guidelines are used for treating workers'

compensation cases in California and a few other states as the basis for approving acupuncture treatments.

Ancillary services: Services rendered in connection with inpatient or outpatient care including medical emergencies that assists but is not part of the main medical service. Can include ambulance service, anesthesiology, pathology, and radiology.

Annual limits: Insurance benefits may be limited, either by a total dollar amount or visit limits. An example would be when acupuncture may be limited to 20 visits per calendar year.

AP: Acupuncture Physician. Legal designation for practitioners licensed in Florida.

Appeals: If an insurance company denies coverage, the practitioner or contractee can appeal this decision. By law, every insurance company must have an appeals process. In addition, if an appeal to the insurance company fails, a complaint may be registered in most states with the state insurance commissioner.

AR: See Accounts Receivables.

Assignment of benefits: A form a patient signs requesting their health benefit payments be made directly to a designated person or facility. This is necessary to receive checks directly from an insurance company for services rendered rather than have them sent to the patient and needing to collect from them.

Audit: In health insurance, an audit is where an insurance company requests records from a practitioner or facility to insure compliance to governmental laws and regulations and insurance company rules.

Authorization: The approval of care from an insurance company. Can be documented on a clinical treatment form.

Back office functions: Back office functions include anything dealing with patient care and include the clinical assistants and practitioner functions. This is in contrast with front office functions.

Basic benefits: Minimum healthcare payments provided under any given health insurance policy.

Benefits: The services an insurance company agrees to cover under an insurance contract.

Birthday rule: This applies to when both parents have insurance that cover a dependent. Some insurance companies use this rule to determine which parent is primary payer. Whichever parent has the earlier month and day of birth, not including the year, is the primary insurance carrier. A court order for one of the parents to be the primary carrier would supersede this rule.

CA: Certified Acupuncturist. License designation in several states such as Montana.

CAB: California Acupuncture Board.

CAM: Complementary and Alternative Medicine.

Capitation: This is a managed care system where a medical provider is paid on a time basis per assigned "head" or patient whether or not the patient actually receives services. For example, under a given contract a doctor may receive $10 per patient per month (PMPM) regardless if they actually see any of the patients assigned by the insurance company. This is how most HMO providers are paid.

Case manager: A nurse at an insurance company, especially within the workers compensation system, that oversees the medical aspects of a claim. Similar to an insurance adjuster but manages the medical side of a claim rather than the administrative aspects.

Center for Medicare/Medicaid Services (CMS): U.S. government office that oversees Medicare and Medicaid. Acupuncture is not part of Medicare, but some states do offer acupuncture as part of their state-administered Medicaid programs. The decisions and edicts of this office have widespread consequences for every healthcare entity and provider.

Certified public accountant (CPA): An individual who has passed a licensing exam in order to provide expertise in oversight of accounting services and tax preparation.

CF: See Conversion Factor.

CHAMPUS: See Civilian Health and Medical Program of the Uniformed Services.

Civilian Health and Medical Program of the Uniformed Services (CHAMPUS): This is the old name for the military and public health service facilities insurance program. The new name is Tricare standard.

Claim: Information submitted by a provider or member in order to receive payment for covered medical services. See CMS 1500 form.

Clinical treatment form: Form documenting authorizations. See authorization.

Closed panels: In certain localities, an insurance company may say that they are no longer adding providers. This means that a provider cannot accept that insurance and get reimbursed in that locality until they are accepted as a provider.

CMS: See Center for Medicare/Medicaid Services.

CMS 1500 form: Center for Medicare/Medicaid Services form. This is the basic form for billing insurance. Used to be called the HCFA 1500 or just HCFA form. The official name for what is more commonly referred to as a claim form.

Copay: The fixed amount the patient pays at time of service. This is deducted from the allowed amount the insurance company will reimburse for services.

COBRA: See Consolidated Omnibus Budget Reconciliation Act of 1985.

Coinsurance: Instead of paying a fixed amount up front as in a copayment, the policyholder must pay a percentage of the insurance's allowed amount. This is considered after the deductible is paid.

Coinsurance limit: This is the limit for how much coinsurance is paid. After this limit is reached, the insurance company pays 100% of the treatment for the remainder of the plan year. Sometimes called out-of-pocket expense.

COB: See coordination of benefits.

Comprehensive insurance: A type of insurance that covers major medical benefits and usually includes most other types of benefits including dental, vision, and CAM.

Computer-based patient record (CPR): Much more than a computerized version of a medical chart, a CPR is a sort of "personal electronic library" providing access to all resources on a patient's health history and insurance information. These are consumer oriented and accessible as opposed to electronic healthcare records (EHRs), which are primarily accessible by medical professionals.

Consolidated Omnibus Budget Reconciliation Act of 1985 (COBRA): An act that includes a provision requiring most employers with group health plans to offer their employees temporary continuation of their health care coverage under their employer's plan if the coverage would stop because of job termination, layoff, or other change in employment status.

Contractee: The primary person on an insurance policy. Same as subscriber.

Conversion factor (CF): This is how much each relative value unit (RVU) is worth in terms of dollars. It is determined by the Centers for Medicare and Medicaid Services based on a formula. In 2008, the CF was $38.087. Over the years this has been reduced and in 2011 is $33.9764

Coordination of benefits (COB): When two or more insurance plans apply to an individual, coordination of benefits means determining which is the primary insurance plan and how the companies will coordinate payment of benefits.

Cosmetic procedure: A procedure performed for the improvement of appearance rather than for medical necessity. When performed secondary to a disfigurement, these procedures may be covered; otherwise they are not generally covered by insurance.

Coverage limits: This is the maximum dollar amount some health plans will pay for health care. The policyholder is usually expected to pay any charges in excess of the health plan's maximum for a specific service. Some plans may have annual or lifetime maximums, which means the policyholder will have to pay any costs above this maximum.

Coverage renewal: The ability to renew insurance coverage at the end of a term, usually one year. By law, insurance coverage cannot be cancelled because of a medical condition. In other words, so long as an individual meets eligibility requirements, coverage must be renewed.

Covered expenses: Medical expenses that are paid for by a given insurance policy. A synonym for benefits and covered services.

Covered services: See Covered Expenses.

CPA: See certified public accountant.

CPR: See Computer-based Patient Record.

CPT codes: See Current Procedural Terminology codes.

CTF: See clinical treatment form.

Current procedural terminology (CPT) code: A 4- or 5-digit code used to describe procedures and modalities performed in clinical settings. These codes are necessary on all claims submitted to an insurance company.

Deductible: The amount that the policy-holder must pay out-of-pocket before the health plan pays its share.

Dependent: An individual related to the primary policyholder who is covered by that insurance policy.

DOB: Date of birth.

DOM: Doctor of Oriental Medicine. License designation for a few states such as New Mexico.

Down-coding: The process of reducing a code from one of a higher value to one of a lesser value resulting in lower reimbursement.

Durable medical equipment: Equipment prescribed by a medical provider which meets the following criteria: it is medically necessary, designed for prolonged use, not primarily or customarily used for nonmedical purposes, and serves a specific therapeutic purpose.

E & M: See Evaluation and Management.

E-codes: Used to classify environmental events, circumstances, and conditions as the cause of a medical condition such as injury or poisoning.

EHR: See Electronic Healthcare Records.

EIN: See Employer Identification Number.

Electronic Healthcare Records (EHR): These are patient records that are kept on the computer. Can be based on a single computer, an onsite network of computers, or based on an internet program. An older but still used term for electronic healthcare records is electronic medical records (EMR).

Employer identification number (EIN): Used instead of social security number for businesses. Legally, it is only needed once you hire employees or are paying yourself as an employee.

EMR: See Electronic Healthcare Records.

Enrollee: The primary person on an insurance policy. Synonyms include subscriber or contractee.

Enrollment date: The initial starting date of coverage in an insurance plan.

EOB: See Explanation of Benefits.

ERISA: Employee Retirement Income Security Act of 1974. This is one of the basic federal laws that regulate medical coverage by employers and other organizations such as unions. Unfortunately, while compliance with this act is necessary, each state has numerous laws that interact with it preventing easy comprehension of the insurance laws.

Evaluation and management (E &M) codes: These are CPT codes that include more than normal history, examination, medical decision making, coordination of benefits, and/or counseling. There are initial E & M codes that are used on the initial visit if they have not been billed in the previous 3 years, or returning E & M codes if the criteria for the initial examination were not met. The normal acupuncture codes indicate a minimal amount of these areas and returning E & M codes cannot be billed too frequently (usually every 4-10 visits).

Exclusions: These are services not covered by insurance. The policyholder is generally expected to pay the full cost of noncovered services.

Experimental: Most insurance companies deny coverage for any procedures or tests which have not been validated by recognized clinical trials. For acupuncturists, with the exception of pain, nausea, and acupuncture anesthesia, most diagnoses are experimental and are regularly denied coverage. Basically, the same as investigational.

Explanation of benefits (EOB): Forms sent by insurance companies to both enrollees and providers providing information about claim payments and what the patient is responsible to pay.

Fee-for-service (FFS): "Traditional" form of insurance where insurer pays a percentage (usually 80%) of fees billed for a procedure. Relatively rare in today's insurance market.

FFS: See Fee-for-Service.

Fiduciary: This refers to a person, acting in a position of trust, who manages funds or benefits for another. They generally are required, by law, to act in the best interests of the beneficiary. Lawyers often fulfill this capacity, especially in personal injury cases.

Flexible spending account (FSA): These are accounts that are contributed before taxes by employers and can be set up to pay for medical expenses. While they cover acupuncture, they may not cover herbs like a health savings account (HSA). A large disadvantage, especially when compared with HSAs, is that the FSA must be spent within a certain time limit, usually one year. These have been supplanted by HSAs and Health Reimbursement Accounts (HRAs).

Formulary: A list of drugs that an insurance company will pay for under a given insurance policy. Drugs not on the list either are not paid for or reimbursement is significantly reduced. While not currently relevant to acupuncturists, maybe, hopefully, herbs may one day be covered and would be part of a formulary.

Front office functions: Front office functions include anything to do with dealing with nonclinical patient needs. These include scheduling, check-in and check-out, and other administrative and customer service functions. This is in contrast with back office functions.

FSA: See Flexible Spending Account.

Gatekeeper: In a managed care system such as a health maintenance organization (HMO), the gatekeeper is the person who is contractually able to refer a patient to a specialist. Usually this is the person's general or family practitioner known as a primary care physician (PCP).

Geographic practice cost index (GPCI): A number that varies by geographical region used to help compute Medicare payments in any given area. For more information and the current figures, please look at: *http://www.cms.hhs.gov/PFSlookup/03_PFS_Document.asp#TopOfPage*.

GPCI: See Geographic Practice Cost Index.

Group health plans: A plan providing health care coverage for employers, student organizations, professional associations, religious organizations, and other groups. This is in contrast to individual, supplemental, medpay, workers compensation, or government plans.

HCFA 1500 form: Healthcare Financing Administration form. This is another, older name for the CMS 1500 (see above).

HDHP: See High Deductible Health Plan.

Health maintenance organization (HMO): A type of managed care plan where an enrollee pays a premium and chooses a primary care physician belonging to the HMO who directs the patient's care. These plans usually offer less freedom when compared to other types of plans, however costs are minimized.

Health reimbursement account (HRA): This is a savings account to which an employer contributes in order to pay some health expenses. It is combined with a high deductible health plan (HPHP). These are very similar to a Health Savings Account (HSA) except in this case the employer rather than the employee pays into it.

Health savings account (HSA): A savings account that has numerous tax advantages and can be used to pay for medical expenses. HSAs are often used in conjunction with a high deductible health plan (HDHP). These are very advantageous to acupuncturists as they are one of two insurance-type products that could potentially pay for herbs.

HIA: Health incentive accounts. These can reward users for living healthy and making healthy choices.

High deductible health plan (HDHP): This is an insurance plan that has a high deductible. It is used in conjunction with health saving accounts (HSA) under the Medicare Prescription Drug, Improvement, and Modernization Act of 2003.

HIPAA: Health Insurance Portability and Accountability Act of 1996. Helps regulate privacy and security of medical information, policy portability, access to coverage, renewability, nondiscrimination, and mandated benefits.

HMO: See Health Maintenance Organization.

HRA: See Health Reimbursement Account.

HSA: See Health Savings Account.

ICD: International Classification of Disease. Often, in the US, followed by a -9 indicating the 9th revision. Codes used for classifying diseases. They consist of 3 digits followed by a decimal and either 1 or 2 digits. These codes are necessary on all claims submitted to an insurance company. For acupuncture, one should always use a code indicating pain. Codes that start with an 8 indicate an accident and should be avoided for insurance billing as they may not pay, indicating that it should be a PI or WC case.

In-network providers: Medical providers, such as acupuncturists, who have a contract with an insurance company to provide and be reimbursed for medical services. Same as a participating or par provider.

Indemnity plans: Plans that reimburse the patient for medical expenses incurred.

Individual plan: Plans sold directly to an individual as opposed to a group plan.

Individual practice association (IPA): Any legal entity that contracts with both medical providers and payors, such as an insurance company. They are often formed by groups of doctors in order to increase reimbursements from insurance companies through collective bargaining.

Insurance adjuster: Individual employed by an insurance company who oversees the processing of an insurance claim. This is a particularly important person within the workers compensation system and when dealing with personal injury cases.

Insurance tracer: A form submitted to an insurance company in order to investigate an outstanding claim. This ability is a right of a medical provider by law.

Investigational: Most insurance companies deny coverage for any procedures or tests which have not been validated by recognized clinical trials. For acupuncturists, with the exception of pain, nausea, and acupuncture anesthesia, most diagnoses are investigational and are regularly denied coverage. Basically, the same as experimental.

IPA: See Individual Practice Association

L.Ac.: Licensed Acupuncturist. A common licensing designation in several states around the nation.

Lien: Used in personal injury cases, this is a contract whereby the individual's attorney promises to pay outstanding medical bills from the case settlement.

Lifetime maximum: The total dollars an insurance policy will pay out over the life of the plan. These amounts are usually very large and have little bearing on acupuncture reimbursement.

Major medical insurance: A type of policy that covers most types of medical expenses.

Managed care: Where certain health insurance companies attempt to influence treatment decisions of healthcare providers in order to increase efficacy and reduce costs. Some of these influences include financial incentives, development of treatment protocols and best practices, and prior authorization of certain services.

MassHealth: Massachusetts's implementation of the federal Medicaid program.

Medical necessity: The basic criteria for insurance coverage in that any procedure performed and submitted for reimbursement must be justifiable, through proper charting and professional standards, in treating a medical condition.

Medical provider network (MPN): In California, MPNs are used to organize medical providers, including acupuncturists, to be part of the worker's compensation system. If a practitioner does not belong to an MPN, it is very difficult for them to see worker's comp patients.

Medical savings account (MSA): A type of plan where individuals could save for medical expenses and achieve tax benefits. The health savings account (HSA) is more beneficial and has supplanted the MSA.

Medicaid: The federal health insurance system covering low income and disabled individuals. While it is substantially funded by the federal government, it is administered by states, which often have their own names for the program. For example, in California, Medicaid is called MediCal.

MediCal: California's implementation of the federal Medicaid program.

Medicare: A federal insurance program that primarily covers individuals over 65 and with certain disabilities. It currently does not cover acupuncture as a treatment modality.

Medicare supplemental insurance: This is an insurance policy that adds benefits to the standard federal Medicare insurance. Rarely, these added benefits include acupuncture.

Med-pay: A type of auto insurance covering medical expenses resulting from an accident It provides coverage regardless of who is at fault.

MIEC: Medical Insurance Exchange of California. A California-based insurance company that provides malpractice insurance to acupuncturists practicing in several states.

Modality: A physical object applied to a body part in order to affect a therapeutic change. If a CPT code is assigned to a modality, it may be reimbursable by insurance.

Modifier: These are codes used to alter a CPT code when circumstances warrant. Examples include taking a shorter or longer time with a given procedure or performing an evaluation at the same time as a procedure.

MPN: See Medical Provider Network.

MSA: See Medical Savings Account.

National provider identifier (NPI): This is a number, mandated by federal law, every individual practitioner and their clinic must have, regardless if they bill insurance. Can be obtained from *https://nppes.cms.hhs.gov*.

NCCAOM: National Certification Commission of Acupuncture and Oriental Medicine. This organization certifies Oriental medical practitioners that have demonstrated minimal training levels and passed certification exams. However certification does not mean licensure, even though certification is the first step to licensure in most states.

No-fault insurance: While this can technically apply to any type of insurance, it most often applies to automobile insurance. In a no-fault situation, claims are paid by the insured's insurance company regardless of who is at fault. Generally, civil lawsuits for recovery are prohibited.

Non-par providers: Medical providers, such as acupuncturists, who do not have a contract with an insurance company to provide and be reimbursed for medical services. Same as an out-of-network or nonparticipating provider.

Nonparticipating providers: Medical providers, such as acupuncturists, who do not have a contract with an insurance company to provide and be reimbursed for medical services. Same as an out-of-network or non-par provider.

NPI: **See National Provider Identifier.** National Provider Identifier. This is number that each individual practitioner must have. In addition, the clinic must have its own unique NPI. Which NPI you use on a claim form (CMS 1500) will depend upon how the insurance company recognizes you (by provider name or clinic name). Can be obtained from *https://nppes.cms.hhs.gov*.

NPPES: National Plan and Provider Enumeration System. Organization that provides the NPI.

Out-of-network providers: Medical providers, such as acupuncturists, who do not have a contract with an insurance company to provide and be reimbursed for medical services. Same as a non-participating or non-par provider.

Out-of-pocket maximums: The opposite of coverage limits, in that the policy-holder's payment obligation ends upon reaching the out-of-pocket maximum, and the health plan pays all further covered costs. These maximums can be limited to a specific benefit category (such as prescription drugs) or can apply to all coverage provided during the year.

Outcome assessments: Calibrated and researched instruments which help determine the progress of a patient with a given chief complaint. These assessments are available for nearly every chief complaint. Examples include: Oswestry Low Back Disability Questionnaire or Hamilton Rating Scale for Depression.

Par providers: Medical providers, such as acupuncturists, who have a contract with an insurance company to provide and be reimbursed for medical services. Same as an in network or participating provider.

Parity laws: A law that states if an insurance company will pay a medical doctor for providing a procedure, they must pay any qualified practitioner for performing the same procedure. For example, California has a parity law, therefore if an insurance company pays a medical doctor to perform acupuncture, they must pay an acupuncturist the same rate for performing acupuncture. Exceptions to these laws are federal insurance programs and self-funded insurance.

Participating providers: Medical providers, such as acupuncturists, who have a contract with an insurance company to provide and be reimbursed for medical services. Same as an in network or par provider.

Patient flow: This is how patients experience the office and includes pre-visit, during the visit, and post-visit aspects. Ideally patient flow shows maximize efficiency and should be a pleasant experience for the patient.

PCP: See Primary Care Physician.

Per-member per-month (PMPM): A plan where patients are assigned to healthcare practitioners and the practitioner is paid a flat monthly fee for each patient whether a patient is not seen at all or is seen every day. A method used to reduce the risk of the insurance carrier and pass some of the risk to the practitioner. The practitioner has the benefit of a steady monthly income though the patient visit load is variable and usually overburdening. Again, primarily seen in HMO environments.

Personal injury (PI): This is a case that involves an accidental injury of some type, such as an automobile or slip-and-fall incident, and often lawyers. PI cases are usually complicated by legal aspects as well as medical aspects. They also involve liens, which mean the acupuncturist may not be paid until the conclusion of the case. Proper charting in these types of cases is absolutely necessary as being called to testify in court is a distinct possibility. Outcome assessments are highly recommended. While having a few open PI cases can be very lucrative for an acupuncture practice, they are much more complicated and time-consuming then an average patient and the acupuncturist should be versed in how to handle them.

PHI: See Protected Health Information.

PHO: See Physician-Hospital Organizations.

PHS: See Public Health Service.

Physician-hospital organizations (PHO): These are organizations established by healthcare providers to increase bargaining power when dealing with managed care companies.

PI: See Personal Injury.

PI Lien See Lien.

PIP: Personal injury protection. Pays for injuries from an automobile accident, same as medpay.

Plan administrator: The company responsible for the day-to-day functions of an insurance plan. They generally process claims and perform other services.

PMPM: See Per-Member Per-Month.

PMS: See Practice Management Software.

Point of service (POS): A type of insurance plan which is a hybrid of a standard HMO plan and a PPO plan. Like an HMO, a client has an in-network primary care provider who is the gatekeeper to specialists and other medical providers. Unlike an HMO and like a PPO, the patient may choose to see any specialist they like (once referred), though there may be some difference in coverage for out of network providers. These plans provide some of the cost savings of an HMO while preserving some of the patient's choices for healthcare.

Policy: This is the contract between the health insurance company and the policyholder which may be an individual or an organization like an employer.

Policyholder: The primary enrollee of an insurance policy. Others may be associated with and covered by the same insurance policy. See dependent.

Portability: The ability to move from one insurance policy to another. This may become an issue when there are pre-existing conditions.

POS: See Point of Service.

Power of Attorney: This a legal document allowing transferring of legal decision powers from one individual to another. While there can be unlimited powers of attorney, these usually and should only be done in cases of *non compos mentis* or "not of sound mind." They may be needed in various legal interactions and in this case they are often limited. For example, in insurance, they will be used to give an attorney the ability to negotiate a personal injury case.

PPO: See Preferred Provider Organization.

Practice management software (PMS): This is software that aids the running or management of a practice. They often include patient and provider scheduling, communication, patient administrative and billing records, insurance billing, and other work flow components. They can be combined with electronic healthcare records (EHR) or electronic medical records (EMR).

Pre-authorization: Authorization for a medical service may be required before admission or care is provided by specialty care providers.

Pre-existing condition: This is when a person has been diagnosed or treated for an illness or medical condition within a specified period of time prior to becoming insured. Often a waiting period must occur before full insurance coverage is operational. A typical waiting period is six months. So, if a patient's covereage began on 01/01/11 and they see you on 02/01/11, the insurance company may question the condition as pre-existing. Coversely, if you saw the patient 08/01/11, pre-existing would probably not be questioned.

Preferred provider: Healthcare providers who are contracted with an insurance company are considered in-network and preferred providers.

Preferred provider organization (PPO): These are networks of healthcare providers that agree to provide services at discounted rates and/or to follow certain utilization rules for patients enrolled in health plans. Typically patients enrolled in a PPO are given incentives to choose in network providers. These incentives may include lower copayments and/or reduced deductibles.

Premium: The amount the policy-holder pays to the health plan each month to purchase health insurance coverage.

Primary care physician (PCP): This individual is the center of the managed care system and determines what care may be necessary for a patient and provides referrals for appropriate services.

Primary insurance carrier: In the case of a patient having multiple insurance policies (say their own, their spouses and/or a supplemental policy), the primary insurance carrier is the one who is billed first and may pay the bulk of the bill.

Primary treating physician (PTP): A physician within the workers compensation system or in a personal injury case who has primary oversight for the patient's medical care. Decisions of medical care usually need to be prescribed or authorized by the primary treating physician.

Prior authorization: See Pre-authorization.

Procedure: A medical service.

Protected health information (PHI): Individually identifiable health information including the patient's name, social security number, date of birth (DOB), telephone number, medical record number, address, and medical records.

PTP: See Primary Treating Physician.

Public health service (PHS): This is the bureaucracy which oversees public health in the United States. It is a primary service under the Department of Health and Human Services and oversees many organizations of the government including the Food and Drug Administration (FDA), Centers for Medicare and Medicaid Services (CMS), the Center for Disease Control (CDC), and the National Institutes of Health (NIH).

QME: Qualified Medical Examiner.

Qualified medical expenses: Medical expenses recognized by federal laws and regulations that can be applied to health savings accounts.

R.Ac.: Registered Acupuncturist. License designation in several states.

Release of information: In insurance, a release must be signed by a patient before disclosing almost any medical information to anyone or entity other than the patient. Exceptions include legal subpoenas, and in cases that fall under mandatory reporting such as abuse or imminent suicide. HIPAA is the main arbiter of how to release information.

Relative value unit (RVU): These units are a number representing the cost for a given procedure or service. There are three components of these costs: physician's work, practice expense, and malpractice costs.

Renewability: Health insurance coverage is usually limited to a one-year duration. Renewability refers to how and under what circumstances the coverage can or cannot be extended to another period of time.

Risk pooling: An underlying principle for the development of all kinds of insurance. The idea is that by gathering many individuals, you can reduce an individual's risk of economic devastation from a catastrophic event and distribute its impact to manageable levels among many. In other words, instead of having to pay a $1,000,000 healthcare bill if an individual is unlucky enough to develop serious cancer, having 100,000 members means that it would only cost $10 for each member. Risk pooling also helps create predictable and stable costs.

RVU: See Relative Value Unit.

Schedule of benefits: Provided to an enrollee specifying the amount of coverage provided and the applicable co-payments, coinsurance, deductibles, and limitations of the policy.

Self-funded: See Self-insured.

Self-insured: Many major corporations hire insurance companies and third-party administrators to manage a health plan or trust that the company funds. This reduces the overall costs of providing insurance for their employees. Generally, state laws do not apply to these plans due to the federal Employee Retirement Income Security Act (ERISA) exemption. This means if a state, such as California, has a parity law, it would not be applicable to self-insured plans.

SOAP: A format for writing chart notes which includes the headings of subjective, objective, assessment, and plan.

SOAPE: A format for writing chart notes which includes the headings of subjective, objective, assessment, plan, and education.

Socialized medicine: A term that has no technical definition, but is often used to mean publicly-funded, government-run healthcare.

SPD: See Summary Plan Description.

SSN: Social Security Number.

Staff model health maintenance organization: A health maintenance organization (HMO) where the medical staff predominantly are hired by and are employees of the HMO rather than contracted physicians. Kaiser Permanente is an example of a staff model HMO.

Subscriber: The primary person on an insurance policy. Same as enrollee or contractee.

Subscription-based medical care: Similar to prepaid dental, prepaid legal, and prepaid vision plans. In the context of health plans, they typically pay for a fixed number of predefined services such as preventive care, hospice care, home visits, etc.

Summary plan description (SPD): ERISA demands an SPD must be provided to employed and covered people. It needs to clearly describe benefits and obligations under the plan, their rights under ERISA, information about how to file a claim, and how to appeal a denial of a claim.

Supplemental insurance: An insurance policy that is used in conjunction with another health plan and may help pay deductibles and co-pays and/or adds coverage for additional services such as prescriptions, dental and optometry. Commonly used with Medicare insurance.

Super bills: Invoices given to a patient to send to the insurance company for reimbursement of a medical expense. They must include the provider's address and tax ID (eventually should be an NPI), the patient's name, diagnosis code (ICD), and procedures performed (CPTs) with charges.

TennCare: Tennessee's implementation of the federal Medicaid program.

Third-party payors: In medicine, a transaction is between a provider and a patient; in other words two parties. When another company, such as an insurance company, pays for the services provided, they are called a third-party payor.

Time of service (TOS): This refers to paying for medical services before or at the time they are provided. In most states, medical providers can offer a TOS discount to their patients.

TIN: Tax Identification number. This is the same as an EIN.

TOS: See Time of Service.

Tracer: See Insurance Tracer.

Tricare: Active duty military insurance program. They do not at this time provide coverage for acupuncture services.

Underwriting: When a potential health insurance client applies for a policy, this is the process of determining whether or not the client should be accepted and at what coverage and premiums.

UR: See Utilization Review.

Usual, customary, & reasonable: These are what an insurance company will reimburse for services rendered. While each individual insurance company will determine what is usual, customary, and reasonable, it should be based on the amount ordinarily charged by most providers of comparable services and supplies in the local area.

Utilization review (UR): A program used in managed care plans to reduce unnecessary medical services. A company employee reviews the necessity, use, appropriateness, efficacy or efficiency of services, procedures, providers, or facilities. They have the ability to facilitate or deny authorizations.

VAS: See Visual Acuity Scale.

Visual acuity scale (VAS): An outcome assessment tool which is any one of several available scales that has been found to be a simple yet effective and relevant determination of pain. Generally considered more powerful than a simple subjective scale of 1-10.

Waiting period: A period of continuous employment an employee must complete before becoming eligible for insurance coverage.

WC: See Workers Compensation.

Worker's compensation (WC): A program, mandated by individual states, that insures employees for accidents occurring through their employment. Some state programs do cover acupuncture (such as California), although most do not.

Appendix D: Resources

Web resources:

www.acu-insurance.com: This book's companion website that includes a blog of up-to-date information about insurance billing in the acupuncture field, tons of resources and forms, FAQs, and information on individual insurance companies. This should be, with complete bias, your first stop for information about insurance billing.

www.ama-assn.org: The website for the American Medical Association (AMA). Since the AMA develops the CPT codes and assigns prices to them, this is where to find the current reimbursement for various CPT codes.

www.cms.hhs.gov: This is the official Centers for Medicare and Medicaid Services website. Any questions relating to Medicare and reimbursement for non-procedural codes should be found here.

www.myreceptionist.com: This website and service allows for low-cost online scheduling and provides a toll free number for patients to call and schedule with a live receptionist who answers the phone with a practice's name.

https://nppes.cms.hhs.gov: This is the website to go to in order to get a National Provider Identifier (NPI) number.

www.officeally.com: A free online insurance billing service and practice management system (PMS) with a low-cost optional electronic healthcare records (EHRs).

www.shawnsteel.com: Mr. Steel is an attorney who specializes in personal injury cases and trains medical providers, especially chiropractors and acupuncturists. His website includes numerous resources and he has an email newsletter that is excellent. He provides an insider's look at how to get paid from lawyers and the legal system.

Appendix E: Reference

Current Procedural Terminology (CPT) Codes

Symbols you may see in these tables:

* Should be used with caution as insurance company may not accept or may require additional documentation.

† Should not be used. Insurance companies consider this a red flag and rarely pay for it and may look closer at all your submissions.

‡ Should be avoided as insurance companies rarely pay acupuncturists for this code.

Evaluation and Management (E&M) Codes

Initial Visit (p.)

Evaluation and Management Codes Initial Visit

Code	History	Exam	Medical Decision Making	Typical Face-to-Face Time (minutes)
99201	Problem-focused	Problem-focused	Straightforward	10
99202	Expanded problem-focused	Expanded problem-focused	Straightforward	20
99203	Detailed	Detailed	Low	30
99204*	Comprehensive	Comprehensive	Moderate	45
99205†	Comprehensive	Comprehensive	High	60

Evaluation and Management Established Patient Codes

Code	History	Exam	Medical Decision Making	Typical Face-to-Face Time (minutes)
99211	Problem-focused	Minimal	Straightforward	5
99212	Problem-focused	Problem-focused	Straightforward	10
99213	Expanded problem-focused	Expanded problem-focused	Low	15
99214*	Detailed	Detailed	Moderate	25
99215†	Comprehensive	Comprehensive	High	40

Acupuncture Procedure Codes

Code	Explanation	Minutes	Units
97810	Acupuncture without electrical stimulation, initial 15 minutes of contact with the patient	15	Single
97811	Acupuncture without electrical stimulation, each additional 15 minutes of contact with the patient, with ***re-insertion of needle(s)*** (emphasis added). Must be used with 97810.	15	Multiple
97813	Acupuncture with electrical stimulation, initial 15 minutes of contact with the patient	15	Single
97814	Acupuncture with electrical stimulation, each additional 15 minutes of contact with the patient, with ***re-insertion of needle(s)*** (emphasis added). Must be used with 97810.	15	Multiple

Other CPT Codes

RVU stands for relative value unit and is used to determine how much should be paid for a given CPT code.

Code	Explanation	Notes	Minutes	Units	RVU
97010	Hot or cold packs applied to one or more areas	Typically not paid by health insurance. It is payable for PI cases.		Single	.17
97012	Mechanical traction to one or more areas	Use when using a device to apply traction		Single	.46
97014	E-stim unattended, to one or more areas			Single	.45
97016	Vasopneumatic devices to one or more areas	Might be used for cupping &/or vibratory massage		Single	.54
97018	Parafin Bath		15	Multiple	.30
97026	Infrared therapy	Use for employing a heat lamp			.17
97110	Therapeutic exercise to develop strength, endurance, range of motion, and/or flexibility*		15	Multiple	.91
97112	Neuromuscular re-education of movement, posture, balance, proprioception for sitting and/or standing activities, and/or kinesthetic sense*		15	Multiple	.95
97124	Therapeutic procedure; massage		15	Multiple	.74
97140#	Manual therapy techniques, for example mobilization/manipulation, manual lymphatic drainage, and manual traction, each 15 minutes	Many acupuncturists use this code instead of 97124 when doing massage as it pays more and can be justified	15	Multiple	.85
97250	Myofascial release	**Only used in the California workers comp system instead of 97140**	15	Multiple	

* These are controversial in that they are generally considered physical therapy codes. In some states, including California, they may fall into an acupuncturist's scope of practice. Since they are controversial, careful documentation is even more important than usual.

\# When using 97140 three things should be noted: what technique is used, location, and time. Of note: In the experience of these Authors, it has been helpful from time to time to add a modifier-59 when billing a 97140 code, for it to be paid.

California Workers' Comp Codes

Code	Instead of
97016 Vibratory Massage	Used when using a massager
97018 Paraffin Wax Bath	
97122 Manual Traction	97124 Massage (Only bill if 97250 doesn't work
97250 Myofascial Release	97140 Manual Therapy Techniques
97780	97810
97781	97813
97250 Myofascial Release	97140 Manual Therapy Techniques

Tests & Measurements CPT Codes

Code	Explanation	Minutes	Units	RVU
81002	Urinalysis nonauto w/o scope		Single	$ 3.60
81025	Urine pregnancy test		Single	$ 8.90
82962	Glucose blood test		Single	$ 3.29
87880	Strep A assay w/optic		Single	$16.88
97750	Physical performance test for measurement (eg. musculoskeletal, functional capacity) with a written report, each 15 mins	15	Multiple	$ .95

* 8xxxx laboratory codes do not have RVUs, just straight Medicare reimbursements. To distinguish these straight dollar amounts, the book includes dollar signs before non-RVU reimbursements.

CPT Modifier Codes

Code	
-21	**Prolonged Evaluation and Management (E & M) Service**
	When face-to-face contact is greater than that usually required for the highest E & M level within a given category. Comment: Should be used rarely as reimbursement is iffy and almost always requires additional documentation. CPT codes 99354 & 99355 should be used for additional E & M services, if services were provided intermittently. Use this modifier for continuous patient contact.
-25	**Significant, Separately Identifiable E & M Service by the Same Physician on the Same Day of a Procedure or Other Service**
	Comment: This modifier should be used when an E & M code is used on the same day as a procedure or another service. Remember that the initial acupuncture codes (97810 & 97813) include a small amount of evaluation and management, therefore E & M CPT codes should only be used on the initial visit and intermittently, as medically necessary, thereafter. If a separate E & M code is used in addition to a procedure such as acupuncture, it must be modified with this modifier.
-50	**Bilateral Procedure**
	If a procedure's description doesn't state it is applied to both sides, this modifier indicates a procedure has been performed bilaterally. Comment: The American Medical Association (AMA) has stated the proper use of this modifier is to apply it on one line with one unit applied to the procedure and reimbursement should then include a bilateral procedure. However, some insurance companies prefer adding the -50 modifier to a second CPT *code*.
-59	**Distinct Procedural Service**
	This modifier states that a procedure is distinct or independent from other services performed on the same day. This can include a separate session or patient encounter, a different procedure, a different site, different injury. Comment: This modifier is used when an acupuncturist bills different therapies used on the same visit. For example, some insurance companies will deny a claim where an acupuncture treatment (97810) is performed at the same time as a manual therapy (97140). If a -59 modifier is used on 97140, it generally goes through with fewer issues.

Appendix F: Bibliography

American Specialty Health. (2006, Aug.). Outcome measurement tools (ver. 6.2). Retrieved May 17, 2008, from Provider Agreement Supplement CD.

California Department of Consumer Affairs Legal Office. (1993, Dec. 13). Legal Opinion No. 93-11. Sacramento: CA.

Claxton, G. (2002, April). *How private insurance works: a primer* [electronic version]. The Henry J. Kaiser Family Foundation.: Menlo Park: CA. Retrieved January 3, 2009 from *http://www.kff.org/insurance/upload/How-Private-Insurance-Works-A-Primer-Report.pdf.*

Cleeland, C. S. & Ryan, K. M. (1994, March). Pain assessment: global use of the Brief Pain Inventory. *Ann Acad Med Singapore.* 23(2):129-38.

Collins, S. A. (2006, March). Choosing the right E & M codes [electronic version]. *Acupuncture Today.* 7(3). Retrieved June 14, 2008 from *http://www.acupuncturetoday.com/mpacms/at/article.php?id=30337.*

Collins, S. A. (2008, October). Fee schedules and charges. *Acupuncture Today.* 9(10): 18.

Collins, S. A. (2009, Sept.). Can you charge for requests for records? [electronic version]. *Acupuncture Today.* 10(9). Retrieved August 22, 2009 from *http://www.acupuncturetoday.com/mpacms/at/issue.php?id=619¤t=true*

CPT Codes. (n.d.). In *CPT code/relative value search.* Retrieved June 21, 2008 from *https://catalog.ama-assn.org/Catalog/cpt/cpt_search.jsp.*

Davidson, M. & Keating, J. (2002, January). A comparison of five low back disability questionnaires: reliability and responsiveness [electronic version]. *Phys Ther.* 82(1):8-24. Retrieved May 10, 2008 from *http://www.physicaltherapyonline.net/cgi/content/abstract/82/1/8http://www.physicaltherapyonline.net/cgi/content/abstract/82/1/8.*

Donald, J. C. (2004). *Insurance billing for CAM providers*. Samsara Publishing, Issaquah, WA.

Eisenberg, D. M., Kessler, R. C., Van Rompay, M. I., Kaptchuk, T. J., Wilkey, S. A., Appel, S., Davis, R. B. (2001, Sept. 4). Perceptions about complementary therapies relative to conventional therapies among adults who use both: results from a national survey. *Ann Intern Med.* 135(5):344-51.

Health insurance. (n.d.) In *Answers.com*. Retrieved January 3, 2009 from *http://www.answers.com/topic/health-insurance*.

Healy, E. (2008, August 19). Re: [PCOM Alumni] Treatment Discounts: no can do [Msg 3]. Message archived at *http://mail.pacific-college.edu/mailman/private/alumni/*.

Hill, E. (2003, Sept.). Understanding when to use the new patient E & M codes [electronic version]. *Family Practice Management*. Retrieved June 21, 2008 from *http://www.aafp.org/fpm/20030900/33unde.html*.

Johnson, D. & Thompson, D. (2007, May 25). How to prove your patients are getting better: collecting and using clinic records [electronic version]. *University of Oklahoma College of Allied Health Department of Rehabilitation Science Fall After-Work Series*. Retrieved May 17, 2008, from *http://moon.ouhsc.edu/dthompso/CDM/outcomes.htm#oswestryhttp://moon.ouhsc.edu/dthompso/CDM/outcomes.htm#oswestry*.

Leavitt, D. H. (ed.). (2003). *Chirocode® deskbook*. Chirocode Institute, Inc. Phoenix.

Mapi Research Institute. (2008). PROQOLID database. *http://www.proqolid.org/*.

National Institutes of Health. (2007, Jan. 17). Pain Intensity Scales [electronic version]. *NIH Pain Consortium*. Retrieved May 17, 2008, from *http://painconsortium.nih.gov/pain_scales/index.html*.

Pain Tools (2008). Retrieved May 17, 2008, from *http://www.painworld.zip.com.au/articles/pain_tools.html*.

Paterson, C. (1996, April 20). Measuring outcomes in primary care: a patient generated measure, MYMOP, compared with the SF-36 health survey [electronic version]. *BMJ*. 312(7037):1016-1020. Retrieved May 10, 2008 from: *http://www.bmj.com/cgi/content/full/312/7037/1016?maxtoshow=&HITS=10&hits=10&RESULTFOR-*

MAT=1&andorexacttitle=and&andorexacttitleabs=and&andorexactfulltext=and&searchid=1&FIRSTINDEX=0&sortspec=relevance&volume=312&firstpage=1016&resourcetype=HWCIT.

Software & Information Industry Association. (2009). *Anti-piracy FAQ*. Retrieved May 9, 2009 from *http://joomlatest.siia.net/index.php?option=com_content&view=article&id=387&Itemid=420.*

Tan, G., Jensen, M. P., Thornby, J. I., & Shanti, B. F. (2004, March) Validation of the brief pain inventory for chronic nonmalignant pain. *The Journal of Pain*. 5(2):133–137.

United States Department of the Treasury Office of Public Affairs. (2008, November 19). *Health savings accounts*. Retrieved January 3, 2009 from *http://www.ustreas.gov/offices/public-affairs/hsa/.*

Index

OTHER BOOKS ON CHINESE MEDICINE AVAILABLE FROM:

BLUE POPPY ENTERPRISES, INC.
Colorado: 1990 North 57th Court, Unit A, Boulder, CO 80301
For ordering 1-800-487-9296 PH. 303-447-8372 FAX 303-245-8362
California: 1725 Monrovia Ave. Unit A4, Costa Mesa, CA 92627
For ordering 1-800-293-6697 PH. 949-270-6511 FAX 949-335-7110
Email: info@bluepoppy.com Website: www.bluepoppy.com

ACUPOINT POCKET REFERENCE
by Bob Flaws
ISBN 0-936185-93-7
ISBN 978-0-936185-93-4

ACUPUNCTURE, CHINESE MEDICINE & HEALTHY WEIGHT LOSS Revised Edition
by Juliette Aiyana, L. Ac.
ISBN 1-891845-61-6
ISBN 978-1-891845-61-1

ACUPUNCTURE & IVF
by Lifang Liang
ISBN 0-891845-24-1
ISBN 978-0-891845-24-6

ACUPUNCTURE FOR STROKE REHABILITATION
Three Decades of Information from China
by Hoy Ping Yee Chan, et al.
ISBN 1-891845-35-7
ISBN 978-1-891845-35-2

ACUPUNCTURE PHYSICAL MEDICINE: An Acupuncture Touchpoint Approach to the Treatment of Chronic Pain, Fatigue, and Stress Disorders
by Mark Seem
ISBN 1-891845-13-6
ISBN 978-1-891845-13-0

AGING & BLOOD STASIS: A New Approach to TCM Geriatrics
by Yan De-xin
ISBN 0-936185-63-6
ISBN 978-0-936185-63-7

AN ACUPUNCTURISTS GUIDE TO MEDICAL RED FLAGS & REFERRALS
by Dr. David Anzaldua, MD
ISBN 1-891845-54-3
ISBN 978-1-891845-54-3

BETTER BREAST HEALTH NATURALLY with CHINESE MEDICINE
by Honora Lee Wolfe & Bob Flaws
ISBN 0-936185-90-2
ISBN 978-0-936185-90-3

BIOMEDICINE: A TEXTBOOK FOR PRACTITIONERS OF ACUPUNCTURE AND ORIENTAL MEDICINE
by Bruce H. Robinson, MD Second Edition
ISBN 1-891845-62-4
ISBN 978-1-891845-62-8

THE BOOK OF JOOK: Chinese Medicinal Porridges
by Bob Flaws
ISBN 0-936185-60-6
ISBN 978-0-936185-60-0

CHANNEL DIVERGENCES Deeper Pathways of the Web
by Miki Shima and Charles Chase
ISBN 1-891845-15-2
ISBN 978-1-891845-15-4

CHINESE MEDICAL OBSTETRICS
by Bob Flaws
ISBN 1-891845-30-6
ISBN 978-1-891845-30-7

CHINESE MEDICAL PALM IS TRY: Your Health in Your Hand
by Zong Xiao-fan & Gary Liscum
ISBN 0-936185-64-3
ISBN 978-0-936185-64-4

CHINESE MEDICAL PSYCHIATRY: A Textbook and Clinical Manual
by Bob Flaws and James Lake, MD
ISBN 1-845891-17-9
ISBN 978-1-845891-17-8

CHINESE MEDICINAL TEAS: Simple, Proven, Folk Formulas for Common Diseases & Promoting Health
by Zong Xiao-fan & Gary Liscum
ISBN 0-936185-76-7
ISBN 978-0-936185-76-7

CHINESE MEDICINAL WINES & ELIXIRS
by Bob Flaws Revised Edition
ISBN 0-936185-58-9
ISBN 978-0-936185-58-3

CHINESE PEDIATRIC MASSAGE THERAPY: A Parent's & Practitioner's Guide to the Prevention & Treatment of Childhood Illness
by Fan Ya-li
ISBN 0-936185-54-6
ISBN 978-0-936185-54-5

CHINESE SCALP ACUPUNCTURE
by Jason Jishun Hao & Linda Lingzhi Hao
ISBN 1-891845-60-8
ISBN 978-1-891845-60-4

CHINESE SELF-MASSAGE THERAPY: The Easy Way to Health
by Fan Ya-li
ISBN 0-936185-74-0
ISBN 978-0-936185-74-3

THE CLASSIC OF DIFFICULTIES: A Translation of the Nan Jing
translation by Bob Flaws
ISBN 1-891845-07-1
ISBN 978-1-891845-07-9

A CLINICIAN'S GUIDE TO USING GRANULE EXTRACTS
by Eric Brand
ISBN 1-891845-51-9
ISBN 978-1-891845-51-2

A COMPENDIUM OF CHINESE MEDICAL MENSTRUAL DISEASES
by Bob Flaws
ISBN 1-891845-31-4
ISBN 978-1-891845-31-4

CONCISE CHINESE MATERIA MEDICA
by Eric Brand and Nigel Wiseman
ISBN 0-912111-82-8
ISBN 978-0-912111-82-7

CONTEMPORARY GYNECOLOGY: An Integrated Chinese-Western Approach
by Lifang Liang
ISBN 1-891845-50-0
ISBN 978-1-891845-50-5

CONTROLLING DIABETES NATURALLY WITH CHINESE MEDICINE
by Lynn Kuchinski
ISBN 0-936185-06-3
ISBN 978-0-936185-06-2

CURING ARTHRITIS NATURALLY WITH CHINESE MEDICINE
by Douglas Frank & Bob Flaws
ISBN 0-936185-87-2
ISBN 978-0-936185-87-3

CURING DEPRESSION NATURALLY WITH CHINESE MEDICINE
by Rosa Schnyer & Bob Flaws
ISBN 0-936185-94-5
ISBN 978-0-936185-94-1

CURING FIBROMYALGIA NATURALLY WITH CHINESE MEDICINE
by Bob Flaws
ISBN 1-891845-09-8
ISBN 978-1-891845-09-3

CURING HAY FEVER NATURALLY WITH CHINESE MEDICINE
by Bob Flaws
ISBN 0-936185-91-0
ISBN 978-0-936185-91-0

CURING HEADACHES NATURALLY WITH CHINESE MEDICINE
by Bob Flaws
ISBN 0-936185-95-3
ISBN 978-0-936185-95-8

CURING IBS NATURALLY WITH CHINESE MEDICINE
by Jane Bean Oberski
ISBN 1-891845-11-X
ISBN 978-1-891845-11-6

CURING INSOMNIA NATURALLY WITH CHINESE MEDICINE
by Bob Flaws
ISBN 0-936185-86-4
ISBN 978-0-936185-86-6

CURING PMS NATURALLY WITH CHINESE MEDICINE
by Bob Flaws
ISBN 0-936185-85-6
ISBN 978-0-936185-85-9

DISEASES OF THE KIDNEY & BLADDER
by Hoy Ping Yee Chan, et al.
ISBN 1-891845-37-3
ISBN 978-1-891845-35-6

THE DIVINE FARMER'S MATERIA MEDICA: A Translation of the Shen Nong Ben Cao
translation by Yang Shouz-zhong
ISBN 0-936185-96-1
ISBN 978-0-936185-96-5

DUI YAO: THE ART OF COMBINING CHINESE HERBAL MEDICINALS
by Philippe Sionneau
ISBN 0-936185-81-3
ISBN 978-0-936185-81-1

ENDOMETRIOSIS, INFERTILITY AND TRADITIONAL CHINESE MEDICINE: A Layperson's Guide
by Bob Flaws
ISBN 0-936185-14-7
ISBN 978-0-936185-14-9

THE ESSENCE OF LIU FENG-WU'S GYNECOLOGY
by Liu Feng-wu, translated by Yang Shou-zhong
ISBN 0-936185-88-0
ISBN 978-0-936185-88-0

EXTRA TREATISES BASED ON INVESTIGATION & INQUIRY: A Translation of Zhu Dan-xi's Ge Zhi Yu Lun
translation by Yang Shou-zhong
ISBN 0-936185-53-8
ISBN 978-0-936185-53-8

FIRE IN THE VALLEY: TCM Diagnosis & Treatment of Vaginal Diseases
by Bob Flaws
ISBN 0-936185-25-2
ISBN 978-0-936185-25-5

FULFILLING THE ESSENCE:
A Handbook of Traditional & Contemporary Treatments for Female Infertility
by Bob Flaws
ISBN 0-936185-48-1
ISBN 978-0-936185-48-4

FU QING-ZHU'S GYNECOLOGY
trans. by Yang Shou-zhong and Liu Da-wei
ISBN 0-936185-35-X
ISBN 978-0-936185-35-4

GOLDEN NEEDLE WANG LE-TING: A 20th Century Master's Approach to Acupuncture
by Yu Hui-chan and Han Fu-ru, trans. by Shuai Xue-zhong
ISBN 0-936185-78-3
ISBN 978-0-936185-78-1

A HANDBOOK OF CHINESE HEMATOLOGY
by Simon Becker
ISBN 1-891845-16-0
ISBN 978-1-891845-16-1

A HANDBOOK OF TCM PATTERNS & THEIR TREATMENTS
Second Edition
by Bob Flaws & Daniel Finney
ISBN 0-936185-70-8
ISBN 978-0-936185-70-5

A HANDBOOK OF TRADITIONAL CHINESE DERMATOLOGY
by Liang Jian-hui, trans. by Zhang Ting-liang & Bob Flaws
ISBN 0-936185-46-5
ISBN 978-0-936185-46-0

A HANDBOOK OF TRADITIONAL CHINESE GYNECOLOGY
by Zhejiang College of TCM, trans. by Zhang Ting-liang & Bob Flaws
ISBN 0-936185-06-6 (4th edit.)
ISBN 978-0-936185-06-4

A HANDBOOK of TCM PEDIATRICS
by Bob Flaws
ISBN 0-936185-72-4
ISBN 978-0-936185-72-9

THE HEART & ESSENCE OF DAN-XI'S METHODS OF TREATMENT
by Xu Dan-xi, trans. by Yang Shou-zhong
ISBN 0-926185-50-3
ISBN 978-0-936185-50-7

HERB TOXICITIES & DRUG INTERACTIONS: A Formula Approach
by Fred Jennes with Bob Flaws
ISBN 1-891845-26-8
ISBN 978-1-891845-26-0

IMPERIAL SECRETS OF HEALTH & LONGEVITY
by Bob Flaws
ISBN 0-936185-51-1
ISBN 978-0-936185-51-4

INSIGHTS OF A SENIOR ACUPUNCTURIST
by Miriam Lee
ISBN 0-936185-33-3
ISBN 978-0-936185-33-0

INTEGRATED PHARMACOLOGY: Combining Modern Pharmacology with Chinese Medicine
by Dr. Greg Sperber with Bob Flaws
ISBN 1-891845-41-1
ISBN 978-0-936185-41-3

INTRODUCTION TO THE USE OF PROCESSED CHINESE MEDICINALS
by Philippe Sionneau
ISBN 0-936185-62-7
ISBN 978-0-936185-62-0

KEEPING YOUR CHILD HEALTHY WITH CHINESE MEDICINE
by Bob Flaws
ISBN 0-936185-71-6
ISBN 978-0-936185-71-2

THE LAKESIDE MASTER'S STUDY OF THE PULSE
by Li Shi-zhen, trans. by Bob Flaws
ISBN 1-891845-01-2
ISBN 978-1-891845-01-7

MANAGING MENOPAUSE NATURALLY WITH CHINESE MEDICINE
by Honora Lee Wolfe
ISBN 0-936185-98-8
ISBN 978-0-936185-98-9

MASTER HUA'S CLASSIC OF THE CENTRAL VISCERA
by Hua Tuo, trans. by Yang Shou-zhong
ISBN 0-936185-43-0
ISBN 978-0-936185-43-9

THE MEDICAL I CHING: Oracle of the Healer Within
by Miki Shima
ISBN 0-936185-38-4
ISBN 978-0-936185-38-5

MENOPAIUSE & CHINESE MEDICINE
by Bob Flaws
ISBN 1-891845-40-3
ISBN 978-1-891845-40-6

MOXIBUSTION: A MODERN CLINICAL HANDBOOK
by Lorraine Wilcox
ISBN 1-891845-49-7
ISBN 978-1-891845-49-9

MOXIBUSTION: THE POWER OF MUGWORT FIRE
by Lorraine Wilcox
ISBN 1-891845-46-2
ISBN 978-1-891845-46-8

A NEW AMERICAN ACUPUNTURE By Mark Seem
ISBN 0-936185-44-9
ISBN 978-0-936185-44-6

PLAYING THE GAME: A Step-by-Step Approach to Accepting Insurance as an Acupuncturist
by Greg Sperber & Tiffany Anderson-Hefner
ISBN 3-131416-11-7
ISBN 978-3-131416-11-7

POCKET ATLAS OF CHINESE MEDICINE
Edited by Marne and Kevin Ergil
ISBN 1-891-845-59-4
ISBN 978-1-891845-59-8

POINTS FOR PROFIT: The Essential Guide to Practice Success for Acupuncturists 5th Fully Edited Edition
by Honora Wolfe with Marilyn Allen
ISBN 1-891845-25-X
ISBN 978-1-891845-25-3

PRINCIPLES OF CHINESE MEDICAL ANDROLOGY: An ntegrated Approach to Male Reproductive and Urological Health
by Bob Damone
ISBN 1-891845-45-4
ISBN 978-1-891845-45-1

PRINCE WEN HUI's COOK: Chinese Dietary Therapy
By Bob Flaws & Honora Wolfe
ISBN 0-912111-05-4
ISBN 978-0-912111-05-6

THE PULSE CLASSIC: A Translation of the Mai Jing
by Wang Shu-he, trans. by Yang Shou-zhong
ISBN 0-936185-75-9
ISBN 978-0-936185-75-0

THE SECRET OF CHINESE PULSE DIAGNOSIS
by Bob Flaws
ISBN 0-936185-67-8
ISBN 978-0-936185-67-5

SECRET SHAOLIN FORMULAS FOR THE TREATMENT OF EXTERNAL INJURY
by De Chan, trans. by Zhang Ting-liang & Bob Flaws
ISBN 0-936185-08-2
ISBN 978-0-936185-08-8

STATEMENTS OF FACT IN TRADITIONAL CHINESE MEDICINE
Revised & Expanded
by Bob Flaws
ISBN 0-936185-52-X
ISBN 978-0-936185-52-1

STICKING TO THE POINT: A Step-by-Step Approach to TCM Acupuncture Therapy 2 Condensed Books
by Bob Flaws & Honora Wolfe
ISBN 1-891845-47-0
ISBN 978-1-891845-47-5

A STUDY OF DAOIST ACUPUNCTURE
by Liu Zheng-cai
ISBN 1-891845-08-X
ISBN 978-1-891845-08-6

THE SUCCESSFUL CHINESE HERBALIST
by Bob Flaws and Honora Lee Wolfe
ISBN 1-891845-29-2
ISBN 978-1-891845-29-1

THE SYSTEMATIC CLASSIC OF ACUPUNCTURE & MOXIBUSTION: A translation of the Jia Yi Jing
by Huang-fu Mi, trans. by Yang Shou-zhong & Charles Chace
ISBN 0-936185-29-5
ISBN 978-0-936185-29-3

THE TAO OF HEALTHY EATING: DIETARY WISDOM ACCORDING TO CHINESE MEDICINE
by Bob Flaws Second Edition
ISBN 0-936185-92-9
ISBN 978-0-936185-92-7

TEACH YOURSELF TO READ MODERN MEDICAL CHINESE
by Bob Flaws
ISBN 0-936185-99-6
ISBN 978-0-936185-99-6

TEST PREP WORKBOOK FOR BASIC TCM THEORY
by Zhong Bai-song
ISBN 1-891845-43-8
ISBN 978-1-891845-43-7

TEST PREP WORKBOOK FOR THE NCCAOM BIOMEDICINE MODULE: Exam Preparation & Study Guide
by Zhong Bai-song
ISBN 1-891845-34-9
ISBN 978-1-891845-34-5

TREATING PEDIATRIC BED-WETTING WITH ACUPUNCTURE & CHINESE MEDICINE
by Robert Helmer
ISBN 1-891845-33-0
ISBN 978-1-891845-33-8

TREATISE on the SPLEEN & STOMACH: A Translation and annotation of Li Dong-yuan's Pi Wei Lun
by Bob Flaws
ISBN 0-936185-41-4
ISBN 978-0-936185-41-5

THE TREATMENT OF CARDIOVASCULAR DISEASES WITH CHINESE MEDICINE
by Simon Becker, Bob Flaws & Robert Casañas, MD
ISBN 1-891845-27-6
ISBN 978-1-891845-27-7

THE TREATMENT OF DIABETES MELLITUS WITH CHINESE MEDICINE
by Bob Flaws, Lynn Kuchinski & Robert Casañas, M.D.
ISBN 1-891845-21-7
ISBN 978-1-891845-21-5

THE TREATMENT OF DISEASE IN TCM, Vol. 1: Diseases of the Head & Face, Including Mental & Emotional Disorders New Edition
by Philippe Sionneau & Lü Gang
ISBN 0-936185-69-4
ISBN 978-0-936185-69-9

THE TREATMENT OF DISEASE IN TCM, Vol. II: Diseases of the Eyes, Ears, Nose, & Throat
by Sionneau & Lü
ISBN 0-936185-73-2
ISBN 978-0-936185-73-6

THE TREATMENT OF DISEASE IN TCM, Vol. III: Diseases of the Mouth, Lips, Tongue, Teeth & Gums
by Sionneau & Lü
ISBN 0-936185-79-1
ISBN 978-0-936185-79-8

THE TREATMENT OF DISEASE IN TCM, Vol IV: Diseases of the Neck, Shoulders, Back, & Limbs
by Phi lippe Sion neau & Lü Gang
ISBN 0-936185-89-9
ISBN 978-0-936185-89-7

THE TREATMENT OF DISEASE IN TCM, Vol V: Diseases of the Chest & Abdomen
by Philippe Sionneau & Lü Gang
ISBN 1-891845-02-0
ISBN 978-1-891845-02-4

THE TREATMENT OF DISEASE IN TCM, Vol VI: Diseases of the Urogential System & Proctology
by Phi lippe Sion neau & Lü Gang
ISBN 1-891845-05-5
ISBN 978-1-891845-05-5

THE TREATMENT OF DISEASE IN TCM, Vol VII: General Symptoms
by Philippe Sion neau & Lü Gang
ISBN 1-891845-14-4
ISBN 978-1-891845-14-7

THE TREATMENT OF EXTERNAL DISEASES WITH ACUPUNCTURE & MOXIBUSTION
by Yan Cui-lan and Zhu Yun-long, trans. by Yang Shou-zhong
ISBN 0-936185-80-5
ISBN 978-0-936185-80-4

THE TREATMENT OF MODERN WESTERN MEDICAL DISEASES WITH CHINESE MEDICINE
by Bob Flaws & Philippe Sionneau
ISBN 1-891845-20-9
ISBN 978-1-891845-20-8

UNDERSTANDING THE DIFFICULT PATIENT: A Guide for Practitioners of Oriental Medicine
by Nancy Bilello, RN, L.ac.
ISBN 1-891845-32-2
ISBN 978-1-891845-32-1

WESTERN PHYSICAL EXAM SKILLS FOR PRACTITIONERS OF ASIAN MEDICINE
by Bruce H. Robinson & Honora Lee Wolfe
ISBN 1-891845-48-9
ISBN 978-1-891845-48-2

YI LIN GAI CUO (Correcting the Errors in the Forest of Medicine)
by Wang Qing-ren
ISBN 1-891845-39-X
ISBN 978-1-891845-39-0

70 ESSENTIAL CHINESE HERBAL FORMULAS
by Bob Flaws
ISBN 0-936185-59-7
ISBN 978-0-936185-59-0

160 ESSENTIAL CHINESE READY-MADE MEDICINES
by Bob Flaws
ISBN 1-891945-12-8
ISBN 978-1-891945-12-3

630 QUESTIONS & ANSWERS ABOUT CHINESE HERBAL MEDICINE:
A Work book & Study Guide
by Bob Flaws
ISBN 1-891845-04-7
ISBN 978-1-891845-04-8

260 ESSENTIAL CHINESE MEDICINALS
by Bob Flaws
ISBN 1-891845-03-9
ISBN 978-1-891845-03-1

750 QUESTIONS & ANSWERS ABOUT ACUPUNCTURE
Exam Preparation & Study Guide
by Fred Jennes
ISBN 1-891845-22-5
ISBN 978-1-891845-22-2